Words of Weedsdom

A memoir about smoking pot, self-discovery, and existentialism

by Cee D

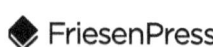 FriesenPress

One Printers Way
Altona, MB R0G 0B0
Canada

www.friesenpress.com

ISBN
978-1-03-915816-0 (Hardcover)
978-1-03-915815-3 (Paperback)
978-1-03-915817-7 (eBook)

1. HEALTH & FITNESS, CANNABIS & CBD

Distributed to the trade by The Ingram Book Company

Table of Contents

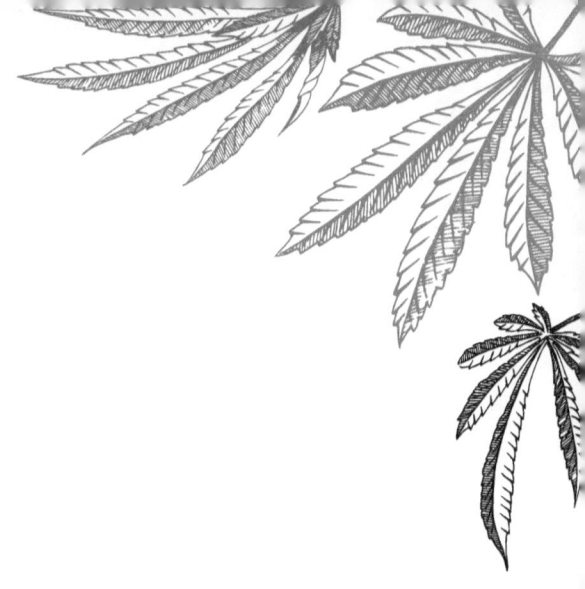

PART I:
BEGINNINGS–
NEW AND OLD

1
Newb

My first experience trying marijuana felt like an inauguration into a cult. My older brother Adam, in his excitement, later admitted to a mutual friend that announcing my desire to try smoking marijuana was one of the coolest things I had ever said. Despite the entirety of our lives that we were related, I was only slightly offended.

On a whim, a date was set for the occasion and at the appointed hour, my sponsors and I convened. In addition to Adam was Jem, my roommate and long-time best friend. These were the two people I trusted most in my life.

Jem and I rented rooms high up in an apartment building surrounded by the busy suburban landscape of Toronto. It was a cozy little bachelorette pad with a panoramic view of the city skyline, accented by a busy bridge under which the subway roared both night and day. The evenings were still warm despite the arrival of the fall season, and city-folk continued to venture out freely without their jackets, stubbornly refusing to acknowledge the loss of another short-lived summer.

Jem's boyfriend Mike had come over earlier (as was his proclivity on Friday nights) and the three of us had been lounging on the couch, chatting aimlessly as we waited for events to unfold. A seasoned cannabis user himself, Mike had been filled in on the evening's plans. Instead of retreating like doves into their nest as they often did, he and Jem waited with me in the living room until my brother arrived.

After a brief knock, Adam entered, removed his shoes at the entrance, and nodded toward the three of us in the corner.

"Sup?" was his standard greeting.

Straight to business, he brandished a slim, white stick from the hidden folds of his hooded jacket. Visions of Popeye candy sticks surfaced in my mind, like gaseous memories from a triggered nostalgia. He offered it to me, outstretched between his thumb and index finger.

"Here you go," he said in his usual monotone voice.

I reached for the proffered joint and plucked it from his grip, rolling it gently between my fingers, intrigued by the delicate feel of the paper. Turning on my heels, I started toward the balcony door before noticing that Jem and Mike had already stood, as if on ceremony. Revealing two of his own smoothly rolled joints in his hand, Mike shrugged.

"I wasn't sure you had your own," he said, indicating that he and Jem had originally intended to share one.

What a gentleman.

Smiling, I mumbled the prerequisite Canadian "thank-yous" before walking to the sliding glass door and tugging on its black plastic handle. Recently repaired by Jem using her MacGyver-worthy skill set, the handle had black string that held the two edges of plastic together. It initially held fast against my pull, but I eventually got it open and led our party out onto the concrete cloud of our balcony.

"The best advice I can give is try not to expect anything," Adam said once we were all outside with the glass door shut snuggly behind us. "I had to smoke a couple times at first before I even noticed anything happening."

He launched into a monologue of his experience as Mike casually handed me a lighter. I paused, hand mid-air in reluctant acceptance; I'd never smoked a day in my life.

"So what do I do, just light it and inhale?" I asked.

"Yeah, light it and suck on it slow, but not too much at once," Jem chimed in for the first time as she brought a cigarette up to her lips.

Although she was trying to quit nicotine, she liked the added flavour when she smoked a joint, making her own chemical cocktail of tranquility. She gently cupped the flame of the lighter to the end of her cigarette with one hand, leaned in to ignite it, and simultaneously drew back with her breath until a small spotlight burned red. Pulling her fingers away from her mouth, she blew out a gentle stream of smoke and nodded to me as I brought my own fingers to my lips with the joint gently perched between them.

I tried to remember how I always saw people do it in movies: holding it gently in their mouths like a pencil and using both hands to cradle the flame as it lights up their face. Or should I pinch it at the end and light it one-handed like Bob Marley might have done? And what should I do with the smoke? Do I inhale to keep it marinating in my mouth, or do I suck it back before it burns the back of my throat and I have to spit it out? Among friends and family, I tried to console myself that I didn't need to play cool. At the very least, I was comforted by the fact that I was in the presence of a very small group of witnesses.

Mimicking Jem, I pinched the joint in my mouth and flicked the lighter at its end with my other hand. The flame quickly grabbed onto the delicate paper and I inhaled slowly, watching as a golden ring began to burn down its length. I felt the smoke as heat invaded my mouth, and although it was not unpleasant, it was quite foreign. I pulled it away, then blew out a steady stream of thick air, releasing it into the night with a guilty sense of pleasure at the conversion of matter. All three witnesses were staring at me. I gingerly held the blunt out to pass it across from me to Mike.

"No," he said. "You always pass to the left."

"Why to the left?" I asked, confused.

"Because. Most people are right-handed, so when you pass to the left they can grab it easier."

I wasn't sure it made sense (was the inconvenience so bad that someone had to make a rule for it? Why discriminate against the lefties?), but my excitement was building. I was being indoctrinated into the secrets of the "Pot-Head" in its natural habitat. Internally, I committed to blend in and surround myself with the customs and beliefs of this culture as an anthropologist might. Despite the lacklustre performance, the deed was done, and I was one of them now.

We continued to pass the ceremonial reefer (in the appropriate manner) around our small circle as we smoked and chatted. I continued in the same way, becoming braver with each round, drawing the golden circle closer to my lips as the smoke ebbed and flowed within my mouth. Adam told us about a trick he and his friends played on each other when they got high. It was called the "Glass Case of Emotion."

For those of you unfamiliar with the concept of 'memes'—a subject very dear to my heart—an explanation is needed. Based on the Greek word *mimema*, referring to something which is imitated, evolutionary biologist Richard Dawkins shortened the word to 'meme.' Likening it to the way cells survive through replication, Dawkins believed that ideas were the same, and that for them to survive they needed to be shared and propagated to remain relevant to society's narrative. Quite simply, 'memes' today refers to humorous images, catchphrases, and scenes in popular media that spread like wildfire throughout the internet community. They are randomly inserted into dialogue to sum up an idea. To a seasoned linguist, a picture may be all that's needed to make a point.

"A Glass Case of Emotion" refers to a scene in the cult classic movie *Anchorman*. The scene depicts Ron Burgundy (a fictional character played by Will Ferrell) crying uncontrollably in a glass telephone booth. While Burgundy's hysterics are in plain sight to those around him, he is silent to the casual onlooker–which makes him look crazy–and the hilarity of the situation is punctuated by the spectators' awkward reactions. This "game" played by my brother and his friends triggers the effects of marijuana's tendency toward paranoia by creating an illusion of sensory deprivation, similar to the spectators watching Burgundy.

Usually done within a small group of people, the trick was best played on an unsuspecting individual.

It begins with an imaginary box. Held between the outstretched hands of the trickster, in mime, a box is placed over an unsuspecting person's head. Once dramatically set down upon the person, the others in the group would begin to have a conversation without sound, moving their lips in casual communication as if nothing strange had happened. I was assured that the results were typically hilarious as the victim would battle internally within their invisible box of silence, and their muddled brain slowly tried to grasp what was (or wasn't) happening. With the drug's tendency to distort perception, the victim would become anxious and for lack of a better term, "freak out", like a grown man having a temper tantrum in public.

I committed this custom to memory as research to consider for later. It seemed juvenile, but maybe that was the point?

As the night drew to a close, I felt no different, much to my disappointment. It seemed as if the monumental change in attitude I underwent to finally try drugs felt wasted (no pun intended). I was a failed experiment. Although nothing seemed lost, nothing was gained. Adam and Jem assured me that what I was experiencing was normal, but this did little to support any optimism I was harbouring—I was aiming too high (pun intended).

With our small torches snuffed and our conversation waning, my admission seemed to mark the end of the congregation. We all shuffled back through the balcony door single-file, toward the warm lights of the apartment. Once inside, Adam headed to his jacket, which was draped messily across the sofa. He reached his hand into one of the inside pockets and pulled out another smoothly rolled joint, which he held out to me. I accepted it from him in a daze, caught up by the strange dèjá-vu.

"You can try it again on your own, maybe when there's less pressure," he said, smiling from the corner of his mouth before throwing his jacket on and shrugging into it. His night was filled with a busy social schedule; he had places to go.

Later that night, with Adam gone and Mike and Jem settled in their lover's nest, I stared at the joint my brother left me. Wondering where to stash it, I decided to tuck it away inside the small drawer underneath my work desk, as if it was a project to continue later. Despite my initial disappointment, I was eager to try again on a practical night—preferably without work the next day. Maybe next weekend, when I had more free time to appreciate the craft. As I considered the pros and cons of an appropriate date and time for my endeavour, slowly my mind succumbed to the lull of traffic from the highway below, and I fell asleep with the soft glow of streetlight on my curtains.

2
Childhood

I grew up in an environment that is common these days. I was very young when my parents divorced, my nuclear family split, and the building blocks of my life were kicked out from under me. With the power of invisibility that comes from being a small child below eye level, I was able to walk into the kitchen of my first family home and see my parents yelling at each other. At that age I didn't understand what was happening— let alone what it meant. I suppose they loved each other once, but there was a mountain of issues I wouldn't come to know until I became much older.

What resulted was a joint custody arrangement. Adam and I lived with our mother most of the time (seven days a week) except for every other weekend when we would visit with our father. The imbalance of time together seemed unfair and this, along with the child support payments, undoubtedly accounted for the bad-mouthing and passive aggressive insults thrown from both sides.

Despite the arrangement we shared with our parents, Adam and I we were not close in our youth. Diagnosed with Tourette's Syndrome and Obsessive-Compulsive Disorder (OCD) after my parent's divorce, my brother scared me. His childhood was challenging, and with a rift in the cheap wood that was used to patch the foundation of our family structure, we all scrambled to keep afloat by keeping the storm-water of his behaviours in balance.

When I tried to interact with him, I would inevitably trigger his volatility (consciously or not, as younger siblings tend to do). I would then trip over myself running to hide in the bathroom—the only room in the house which had a lock on the door. I don't know if he would have ever actually hurt me, but my fear of him resulted in a relationship similar to being a student on a field trip: aware of the expectations, but too distracted to really pay attention. I knew he needed help from my parents, and although I loved him because he was family, I didn't actually know him.

The attention Adam needed was divided as a result of the separation between my parents. I saw the difficulties this presented first-hand, watching in the invisible way that I did. Although my dad was still voluntarily involved in our upbringing, due to our custody situation, Mom was our main caregiver. Being fiercely independent in nature as she was, I don't think my dad ever really knew the extent of our struggles—Mom was too proud to ask for help. She tried her best to find treatment that would help counteract Adam's rages, difficulty concentrating, and self-confidence issues, which resulted in a barrage of medications that numbed him, made him gain weight, and put him through the darkest times of his life. As we got older, we learned more about each other and the childhood we experienced separately. I've only just begun to understand what he went through, but he told me how much he felt like a guinea pig from all the trial and error.

Around the time I was in grade seven and Adam was fifteen, the decision was made to send him to a farm on the outskirts of the city which specialized in working with children with behavioural difficulties. It wasn't a farm in the literal sense (much to my disappointment), and children would often stay there for weeks to months at a time in cabins, performing general labour duties alongside counsellors. Activities were designed to generate structure and discipline, and various classes would supplement the chores of the days, including general public school education and more practical ones, such as woodshop. Every other weekend my mother and I would go to visit Adam, and it was extremely uncomfortable, like visiting a relative in prison.

It was a long drive out of the city, marked in time by the increase of open fields seen through my car window. Whenever I drove with my dad, the radio would always be on to fill the space with Billy Joel, The Beatles, Chicago, The Beach Boys, Roy Orbison, and other 'Golden Oldies.' The silence between us was of our mutual appreciation for the music (although neither my dad nor I were big talkers), and we often shared our moments together comfortably in this way. Whenever I drove with my mom, we never listened to the radio and often sat in silence. Either way, I was soothed by the listless movement from the inside of a vehicle, watching the changing landscapes around me. Perhaps it was a learned habit from existing in the womb while my mom was always on the road for her job in sales.

After nearly two hours of quiet on the road to visit my brother, my mom and I would pull onto a small gravelled road which forged a straight path between two fenced areas. The fences were short, seemingly to enclose something at some point, but now they were empty with large, virgin expanses of untouched grass. We parked next to the main building, situated centrally among the recreational workshops for the students and the small residential cabins. It was a large space with only a handful of people about at any given time, and anyone who saw us pull up always eyed us suspiciously.

With our faces downcast at the shoddy wooden stairs beneath us, we always entered through the main building. Sometimes we were recognized by the staff inside, but often it was someone new that greeted us, and their faces would relax in recognition at the mention of my brother's name, knowing we had reason to be there. Adam usually came and found us standing alongside the entranceway. Although his demeanour remained neutral toward us, I could feel my mother relax beside me as she embraced him, releasing the anxiety she held during the car ride up. I would hug him too, in the detached way I was accustomed to.

We spent most of the day together, with Adam showing us around the farm, talking about what he was made to do and the general routine of the days. His tics would be in full display, the most recent of which was swinging his neck from side to side and touching each ear to his shoulder in a rhythmic motion that sought an invisible sense of symmetry. An old familiar one was also present: rubbing the fingers on his right hand harshly against themselves, mimicking the contractures of a stroke survivor. He was unable to contain the pull his tics had over him, and this was especially the case in stressful times.

My mother and I began our goodbyes once the sun began to set, and again we exchanged hugs. These were the most difficult moments, when Adam would always ask when he could come home. Sometimes he cried in desperation, while other times he was solemn. The extremes of my brother's behaviours haunted my mother, but they always strengthened her resolve to make him stay to get the help he needed. Long accustomed to keeping an emotional distance from him, I played my part as the sister and as the daughter. I remained outwardly supportive but detached to the scenes around me. Truthfully, I was just happy that I didn't need my brother's permission to go into his room and play his video games now.

Unfortunately, I too was later diagnosed with Tourette's Syndrome. Even though my tics were usually more subtle and easier to hide than Adam's, my parents picked up on them as they began to manifest. They began as small noises from the back of my throat, eventually moving to small twitches in the face— usually involving the eyes. As good as I was at staying silent, they would eventually surpass my level of self-control. Like most things, the media's depiction of this disorder is exaggerated and only accounts for a very small percentage of those with extreme symptoms. It may be a punchline for someone to unexpectedly swear or shout vulgarities, but I can assure you, it's more insidious. Like Poe's *Tell-Tale Heart*, the thought of a noise or a movement arises and becomes a force which only you can hear. Then comes a craving to release a sound or gesture that you try to fight hopelessly until you can't take it anymore. A blink, a throaty squeal, a smack of the lips; these small movements mean nothing, and serve no purpose except to embarrass you and harass the mind.

Perfecting my powers of invisibility to deal with my parent's divorce alongside a fear of my sibling, my new medical diagnosis threatened to undo me. I tried to remain inconspicuous by developing a self-imposed isolation, and I was hesitant to form new relationships or open up to anyone. In public school, my tics were impossible for other kids to ignore, and I was eager to dismiss the curious faces with their lack of tact so I could once again hide into the background. Somehow, I was able to convince a group of girls that the small squeaks that emerged every few minutes from my throat were something I did for fun. For a small period of time they bought it, taking cues and participating in the odd ritual from my glitched mind. Eventually, they grew bored, as children often do, and thankfully fucked off.

After my Tourette's diagnosis, my mom took me to see a specialized child psychiatrist, just like she did for Adam. My psychiatrist would get me to draw (something about allowing a child to express how they feel creatively when they aren't able to do so vocally). I was asked to draw simple things, and as I drew she would ask simple questions to push at my defences.

"How is school?"

"How are you feeling?"

Even though these seemed like harmless questions, I refused to answer, preferring instead to maintain a vow of silence and a position of ignorance, focusing instead on my drawings. The next time I went, I wasn't allowed the distraction, and the drawings were gone while the questions remained. For whatever reason, I refused to break. Immune to its awkward nature, I maintained my quietness instead while I waited for it to be over.

Even though I practiced hard to silence my voice, writing seemed to be more my style. In public school French class, after I finished writing a test, some unconscious part of me decided to flip the papers over and pour my soul out on the back of the pages:

Nobody likes me.
I have no real friends.
I'm stupid.
I'm trouble for my parents.
I hate my life.

When it was time to turn the tests in, I remember looking up to see the student beside me looking at me in confusion.

"Why did you write that?" they asked me, but I was silent as always.

Even though their brows were furrowed in confusion, there was an absence of judgement in those eyes, but the attention made me suddenly uncomfortable.

Of course the teacher saw it. I don't know why I would have thought otherwise. I was called one day into the principal's office with my mom and my French teacher, and on the desk was a photocopy of the back of my test with my statements written out. I had written them curved like rainbows down the length of the page, like some silly attempt to blunt their disturbing nature, and now they were exposed to everyone I wanted to hide them from. I remember nothing of what was said in that meeting, but I know nothing changed afterwards. The next time I saw that paper was at home on the living room table, tucked against the stairs, where my mom put documents she needed but didn't have time to sort through. Once I saw it, I immediately grabbed it and tore it to pieces before throwing it into the garbage, trying to erase its very existence.

I saw the effort it required of my mother to look after my brother and I in all aspects (physically, emotionally, and financially), and I was very aware of the amount of attention my brother needed from her. She always looked exhausted to me, yet seeming tireless. Everything she did was for us, as her children.

On any regular day, after working her full-time day job in sales and fundraising, the sound of my mom's keys tinkled in the back door of our townhouse, alerting me to her arrival. The pressure exchanged by the door's opening would disrupt the stagnant air in the house, often followed by the shuffling sound of boxes being brought onto the door-step—hauled in one-by-one—each punctuated by the low click of her heels on the tiled floor. She enjoyed her job, and her social nature made it easy for her to develop strong relationships with her clients. She was always bringing home boxes full of brochures, catalogues, and choco-lates to sweeten her exchanges or prepare for any potential deals.

I was usually up in my room with America's favourite babysitter, the television, planted sixteen inches in front of it (my vision was awful), and focused on the worlds of fantasy it conjured. I loved to watch Sailor Moon as she battled galactic foes alongside her planetary friends or Ash Ketchum's journey across Japan to catch *all* the Pokémon. When my mom came home, I was midway through the first TV show of my back-to-back after-school lineup as I listened to her climbing up the stairs on her stockinged feet.

She went to her room at the top of the stairs, the smallest of the three, and closed the door wordlessly behind her. Although she occu-pied the master bedroom for years, when Adam entered high-school, she graciously switched spaces with him to accommodate for the friends he had over to play video games with for hours at a time.

I heard the soft shuffle of her movements behind the thin wall and the squeak of metal hangers pushed out of the way, and I pictured her searching for the white dress shirt and black apron that she wore for her second job as a waitress at a seafood restaurant. Soft clinking, the sounds of drawers opening and closing, and the door opened again as she made her way to the bathroom at the end of the hall. If she had time, she took a shower before she changed, but usually she just coiffed clumsily, and the sound of the blow dryer would echo off the porcelain of the sink as she dropped it a couple times before she finished.

On her way out of the bathroom, she knocked softly on my door, opening it an inch before I had time to answer, as she always did. I heard the same speech three times a week: she was going to work, could Adam and I please do the dishes that were in the sink? I would reluctantly pull my eyes away from the television screen long enough to make eye contact with her, nod, and assure her we would. When I reminded Adam, he barely acknowledged me—his eyes stayed glued to the screen of his video games—and when I pushed, he yelled. Not wanting to do them myself, they rarely got done.

Her entrance into the house when she arrived home in the evening was more muted. Now in bed, I was weighed down by the guilt, and I pictured her sighing, silent in her disappointment, as she turned on the kitchen taps to fill the sink. The rush of water would echo through the pipes, pawing dully against my ear on the pillow.

In separated families, it's not uncommon for children to adopt the role of a caregiver as a behavioural strategy to try and keep the frayed social ties together. Since I was hyper-vigilant to the vulnerabilities of my mom and Adam, I made a conscious effort as a child to be seen (if necessary) and not heard (an old English dream amiright?). If I stayed quiet and out of the way, I figured Adam would get the attention he needed, and my mom wouldn't have to further exhaust herself with my half. I used a faulty caregiving strategy to ignore my own needs in favour of others'. I was never bitter about it, I just rationalized that my self-neglect was necessary to keep my family together.

I wish I knew then what I finally realize now; that's fucked.

3
Second Time Around

Each evening following my first attempt at smoking cannabis, my thoughts would often find their way to the joint secretly stashed in the drawer of my writing desk at home. Only a couple of days passed before I decided to try again. With Jem and Adam present during my first attempt, I got over my initial fear of dying from trying drugs for the first time. As the sun set earlier these days, I felt that it would work as an appropriate background to shroud my illicit activities on the balcony outside my apartment.

Collecting the joint from its hiding place, I held it delicately between my fingers and borrowed Jem's lighter from the small table beside the balcony door. Gathering a light coat and a pair of boots, I stepped out into the darkness. Even though we overlooked one of the main highways out of the city, the cars below were few and far between, which seemed strange for the Friday I had chosen. Despite the stillness, I noticed that the night was pleasantly warm as I unfolded my camping chair and sat down.

Lighting the end of the joint with Jem's lighter, I pulled softly on its back end, dragging the smoke into the back of my throat like I learned to, and once it began to burn the inside of my mouth, I blew out a steady stream of smoke. I took my time experimenting with the amount of fresh air I brought into my mouth as I inhaled, and how hard I pulled on the drag.

It was about halfway through when I remembered I had left the stove on to heat up my dinner: a frozen pizza. Sitting up quickly, I reached for the handle of the balcony door and felt the ground sway beneath me like I was on a boat in the middle of the ocean. I struggled to control my balance as my brain panicked. I tried to remember how to control one leg at a time to navigate the small step indoors. I finally dropped my feet inside—heavily—and looked around my living room in a daze.

My mind was alive and running the code of *The Matrix*, and I scanned the room as if I had downloaded some kind of Ikea instruction manual, inventorying all pieces before construction.

I was keenly aware of one thought: this was *nothing* like alcohol.

I had become the princess and the pea, feeling even the smallest sensations, and I began an intimate connection with time as everything seemed to slow down around me. As I swayed into my kitchen, I felt the precision of each movement my body made, from the way my mind connected to each of my muscles, to the size and strength of each. I was acutely aware of the concept of balance, but much like my recent challenge with the balcony, it was something that required time to process.

Thoughts bounced around inside my skull, kicked into fast-forward, which was strange considering how slowly time seemed to move around me. The simplest of tasks caused an intense internal experience, but my body moved at a glacial pace. I felt aware of everything, and every sound, smell, and movement triggered my consciousness like a factory hard-wired for efficiency. I felt detached from reality as one does when intoxicated with alcohol, yet still in possession of my every thought and movement.

Opening the door of the refrigerator, I peered inside, but as a mass of gyrating human flesh, bone, and sinew, I ultimately forgot what I was doing there. I was too focused on this new experience, thinking *this* must be what I was supposed to feel the first time. *This* is what it was to be high.

It was a while before I noticed the light on the stove, which triggered the memory of my dinner. My body wasn't hungry anymore, but my mind craved new things to puzzle over, process, and consume. I was like a ball of yarn needing to untangle itself. Absentmindedly, I turned the stove off, ignoring my overcooked pizza for now.

Jem and I had recently moved into our apartment at the outskirts of a busy Toronto neighbourhood. As I walked from room to room like the cyborg in *Terminator,* I too was composed half of flesh, and half of mechanical purpose. Tapping into a pre-written code to organize and unpack my belongings, I ran my eyes over the labelled boxes of flotsam and jetsam around me. Following new creative inspiration, I began to process the thoughts that sprang forward once I settled on an object.

Where did it all belong? Where should it all belong?

What room had the appropriate amount of items that I wanted to move around?

I lingered just as long as it took to get an idea of what I was dealing with by scanning each object up and down and following the steady stream of input running across my brain like commands in a computer program. Like a goldfish, I was limited by my attention span and frequently found myself going in circles, only to be caught up once again by the current of the infinity-loop layout of my apartment.

I could practically feel the high latching onto any available ports in my brain, leading me through this physical space as a starship commander inside my flesh-suit shell. Eventually (like most stoners), I found myself back in the kitchen. Hunger had become the driving force of my actions, and my meat machine needed to recharge its battery. It was a strange awareness—allowing myself to be driven by pure sensation instead of my usual need for control. The baser needs of my soul took over and opened doors into the unconscious parts of my mind, and these doors would unlock the floodgates to future revelations.

4
Growing Pains

After my parent's separation, my mom, Adam, and I moved farther east into the city, while my dad bought a townhouse just a couple streets away from our short-lived family home. When I visited him, I got to return to the neighbourhood I lived in before my world had changed. Every other weekend I travelled back there, which allowed me to regain a sense of freedom that seemed lost. It was strange having a new room in a new house, but I could tell my dad put a lot of effort into making the rooms for Adam and I, and these days I can appreciate the sentiment behind it, though I didn't recognize it at the time. Even though he and Mom split, the love for Adam and I was palpable through this gesture in the way of a warm welcome saying "I love you, and I tried to make things just the way you like them because I couldn't imagine you two not being in my life."

My fondest memories still exist around my dad's house on Harris Way. In the way fathers tend to be the less paranoid parent, I was allowed to go out on my bike and ride around the neighbourhood all day, as long as I respected the semi-regular check-ins that were tentatively enforced. I added to the mental maps of the neighbourhood I had before my parents separated, and explored the lines and crossings of each street. By the end of each summer, I recognized the growing landscape like the back of my hand.

My regular route rode parallel to the train tracks that were behind my dad's house, past a small bridge with the big letters "CN" painted on it (for the Canadian National Railway) to the small strip-mall behind. This was my usual pit stop; a little reservation I could check into and spend my time practicing capitalism by exchanging candy for my allowance money. My dad, Adam, and I would often take short drives here to get groceries from the Longos grocery store, the *Toronto Sun* newspaper from the convenience store, or a slice of pizza from Pizza Pizza. When a What-a-Bagel opened on the tail-end of the building next to a family restaurant, we often made special trips together to get hot, fresh bagels straight off the conveyor belt and bite into their fluffy, warm innards. When I came by myself sans chaperone, it felt all the more exciting—like I was Harrison Ford's character Deckard in *Blade Runner,* navigating a busy foreign marketplace on a reconnaissance mission. My mission (which I always chose to accept) was to eat an entire bag of garlic sticks on my own before I made it home.

For entertainment, the three of us went to the Video 99 in the mall to rent movies on VHS tape. There was a popcorn cart in the middle of the store that was free for customers. With my powers of child invisibility, I often filled up a small bag and ventured to the "adult section," which was partitioned off to the east side of the store by a small curtain that never stayed closed. It became a ritual to sneak a peek behind the curtain to see if anyone was back there (sometimes there were men, but they were always alone), and when there wasn't, I looked curiously at all the pictures of naked women, seemingly surprised and doing gymnastics, while I crunched on my popcorn.

Although my mom ensured Adam and I followed through with the visits to Dad's when they were expected, when we reached our teenage years, we were no longer obligated to. When he wasn't required, Adam refused to go, but whether this was because of the strained relationship he had with our dad, or because of the behavioural issues that followed him into adolescence, I don't know. I continued to visit because of the possibility for adventure, and the focused attention of my dad.

My adolescence wasn't markedly different from my childhood. Generally speaking, the teenage years are defined by a mixture of curiosity, angst, egocentrism, and a strong need for independence. Given the subject matter of my earlier years, I was ahead of the curve, so my serious nature translated into more of the same as a teen. I thought I knew better than everyone else—pretentious as a result of my experience—and I had been doing everything by myself (or trying to) for years already. I didn't feel the need to rebel against my parents; I already separated myself from them. I didn't feel the need to conform to peer pressure to make many friends; I was comfortable in my independence, and with Jem, who was the exception. Since we met and lived close to one another during our formative years, when the weather was nice (a rarity in Southern Ontario), Jem and I were usually together, but the times when her mother would let her leave the house or allow her friends over were sparse, and I often spent my time doing solitary hobbies.

My main hobby was playing video games, and I lived vicariously through the interactive stories like I did with TV shows and movies. One of my first assertive flexes as a kid was whining to my brother about how I wanted to play the game he was currently playing on his Super Nintendo. Adam also played lots of video games growing up, and he was usually docile when he played, which made me feel comfortable to sit beside him and watch the screen. He was playing the beginning of my now favourite game, *Chrono Trigger*: a cult classic in Japanese role-playing games (JRPGs). You start as the main protagonist who goes to a festival by his house, and to progress, you play carnival games like betting on the winner of a race, "hitting" a puck hard enough (pressing a button on the controller at the right time) to hit a bell, and a version of the Shell game which has you guessing the correct character after several of them shuffle places. As Adam led his red-haired sprite through the screen, my excitement grew, and after annoying him enough trying to convince him to let me play, he started to yell at me. My mom, who was downstairs, yelled back.

"Adam, let your sister have a turn!"

"It's *my* game, I'm still playing!" he yelled back to her.

The exchange between them lasted a few moments, but I eventually cowered into silence by his stubbornness and my mom's lack of follow-through on the matter. I continued to watch him and bide my time. Later, when he wasn't home, I snuck back into his room, turned on the system in the way he did when I watched him earlier, and played the game myself. When I was done, the trick was to leave everything where I found it initially. I was good at leaving no trace of my presence.

When my grandfather passed away from a stroke complication, my dad sold his home on Harris Way and moved in with my Nonna, who was now alone in the family house he and my uncle grew up in. Family dynamics changed for me once again, and although I continued my bi-weekly visits, my adventures came to a halt. The unfamiliar neighbour-hood of my Nonna's house was intimidating and dangerous due to its proximity to the main roads, so my usual outings were more strictly enforced. Now, when I wasn't playing video games at my mom's, I was watching movies at my dad's. I rarely ventured outside when I visited any more, instead holing myself up in the basement and watching mara-thons of my dad's extensive VHS movie collection.

Every so often my Nonna would come down to try and offer me food—which I graciously declined—but you can never say no to food from an Italian grandmother, so it was later forced into my proximity whether I wanted it or not.. My dad would occasionally come downstairs and attempt to have a conversation with me, but even these were inter-ruptions I grew to hate, despite watching a movie I had seen dozens of times before.

Despite the limited interaction, I enjoyed visiting him. Our natures were similar enough to be comfortable in our own company, but there was always a shyness that was hard to express, which made it difficult to impose on the other. I was habitually quiet and avoided attention, but when I was in a receptive mood, we ventured out to see a movie in the the-atres or went to a store to buy something I had my eye on. Because of this, our time together often became one of proximity with little interaction.

5
Loneliness And Love

For all intents and purposes, I chose to be alone, but that doesn't mean I wasn't lonely. Love and caregiving were synonymous to me because I grew up watching how my mom needed to be there for Adam. Caring for others looked like hard work, and from childhood I convinced myself that there were those who needed love before me, like Adam did. Escaping reality was something I practiced growing up through TV and movies. I was fed fantasy with Disney as my wet nurse, drawn into the romance of the imaginary and guaranteed happy endings. I was placated by stories of love defying all bounds, destiny, and good conquering evil. With the turmoil surrounding my familial love, the romantic love shown to me through popular media seemed like a good alternative.

The term "soulmate" comes from an idea from Plato, who proposed that humans once existed as two beings joined to one another—with four arms and four legs—and were split by the Gods out of wrath, fated to live life forever searching for their other half. This "other half" is a partner who literally completes another, as the other half of a whole being. I became obsessed with this idea. Despite the comfort I found in my own company, I wanted to be in a partnership, and I felt like I would never truly be able to be myself unless I had this validation through someone else.

The desire for a partner to fulfil all my needs as a lover, a friend, or a mentor penetrated every fibre of my being, albeit craftily tucked away through my attempts to stay invisible. On one hand, my desire was to keep my head down and stay small like I'd always done, and on the other, if I had to let someone in, I wanted it to be The One. I wanted a person to fulfil my every need so that I didn't have to expose too much of myself. Initially, this person was supposed to put together all the pieces of my illusive happiness, but ultimately became a scapegoat to hoist all my future dreams upon.

Self-taught by a life of Disney, romance novels, and movies like *The Notebook*, I suppose my immersion into film and television contributed to the fact that I was always crushing over someone in the spotlight. Memories of my life are often delineated through my *savour du mois* (my celebrity crush at the time).

Jim Carrey was my very first celebrity crush. From him, I moved agelessly (and in no particular order) through the likes of Johnny Depp, Nathan Filli(yum), Richard Armitage, Robert Pattinson, Michael Fass(bend me ov)er, and Elijah Wood. I guess you could say I have an obsessive personality and, like a drug addict, I moved from fix to fix. Each crush would invade my brain like a parasite and take over for months, and sometimes years.

I latched onto a celebrity crush and pined over them for weeks at a time. I looked up everything to do with them from their interests and desires to their astrological compatibility with me. I searched for every interview, movie, picture, or piece of information I could about them and created a universe in my head where we were destined to meet like some Hallmark love story. I was part of that awkward culture of fandom that cheers from the audience when they find out their favourite celebrity crush is still single as if, regardless of their current partners, families, or lives, they would ever have a chance.

It was the fairy tales that did me in; the ones where two people come together despite all the odds. I blame Cinderella for making me cling to the idea that those in an elevated social status are the ones I want. I was entirely delusional, but it gave my mind something to distract it from my very real loneliness. Despite any number of male celebrity obsessions I threw in, the black hole that was my love life remained ever present. In all the love stories, the more star-crossed the lovers were, the more romantic it was, and it was nearly impossible for me to ignore the pull toward this delusion.

The search for a mate is the search for what we desire. Plato's idea of soulmates proposes that what we find in our partners is what's missing in ourselves, so that together, we can be whole. How lovely would it be if you were one out of millions of people, that was perfectly suited to another? Unfortunately, these ideals can be a bit dramatic and, quite frankly, unrealistic. It's uncommon to be charismatic when you try to express a feeling, unless you're a practiced poet (or really good at improv). It's not easy to say what you really want without holding back, especially when you're at risk of hurting someone's feelings. Real life is not usually as romantic as Hollywood tries to make us believe.

Ironically, in a heavily populated area it's hard to connect with people, and the dating scene is the opposite of alluring. In a bustling city people have busy lives, and the search for a mate seems rushed and superficial. The club scene can be fun for the weekend, but generally you won't find the pick of the litter behind a bar—not to mention it's impossible to have a conversation with someone over loud, pumping music. Women are no longer the demure, passive creatures of the past, and they can dress confidently in outfits that show off more than their ankles. I had a handicap: growing up as I did by hiding in the shadows. When such overt sexuality attracts mates, I baulked, preferring instead to let the vultures prey, hoping it would thin the herd to reveal someone who was waiting for me the whole time. I didn't know how to market myself.

Sitting at home, lusting over the manicured perfection of an attractive human being across the world from you, all while in the comfort of your own home, is much easier than rejection. Fantasies can never disappoint you in the way reality can. It's a comfortable, (mostly) harmless obsession you can play out in your head, keeping All-American hunk Chris Pine in the back of your mind when you've had a tough day, knowing you can boot up your computer and see his beautiful blue eyes looking back at you through the screen. In addition, having Ryan Gosling innocently stare out at you from your computer, saying, "Hey girl, I know you had a rough day, so grab some wine and come watch me take my shirt off," works just as well.

Why settle for reality when you can play out fantasies safely from the confines of your own mind? I spent a lifetime perfecting invisibility, and old habits die hard.

6

Old Feelings

After high school, I followed an education into health care, where the habits of my childhood followed me into adulthood. I chose nursing out of a desire to help others, and the familiarity of ignoring my own needs. Despite my good intentions, it's no wonder the profession ate me alive.

Putting the needs of others before yourself is one thing if it's for family, but it's another thing in an increasingly challenging health care system where demand dwarfs supply and resilience is needed. I was running on fumes since the start. I missed my breaks often and went hungry more times than I can count to complete the never-ending tasks required of patient care. I held my bladder to the point where my body considered its safety compromised, and conveniently forgot the urge in order to conserve fluids. At some point, every nurse feels shame over their bodily needs, wishing there was more they could do despite working themselves to the breaking point. Self-sacrifice is basically a commandment of the profession, and nurses are unable to refuse assignments, even if their safety is at risk. If we're lucky, we can get support from others, but it never exempts us from entering harm's way to provide treatment, and the idea of putting yourself first often constitutes professional negligence.

It's almost a rite of passage to care for a patient with Clostridium difficile, or C. Diff for short, (a tenacious bacterial infection of the gut which usually results in uncontrollable diarrhea) and, as a new graduate, my time came. Even those fully capable of taking themselves to the washroom can be at the mercy of this disease and promptly shit their pants. It's an awful situation, but what was worse was that the patient I had was non-verbal, requiring what we call in the biz "total care," meaning she couldn't take care of her basic needs in any shape or form. Her diarrhea was relentless, and I couldn't get far into cleaning and changing her before having to start over. It was an exercise in futility.

At the end of an eight-hour shift feeding, washing, and getting patients in and out of bed for appointments or back and forth to the washroom, I was exhausted, and yet every time I walked by this patient's room there was the unmistakable smell of another bowel movement. Even though my shift was nearly over, there was still so much that needed to be done and patients seem to have a sixth sense surrounding shift change, deciding they are suddenly desperate for your attention. I was still so tired, and the smell angered me. Hadn't I done enough? Couldn't the next shift deal with it?

I actively avoided her room. Out of sight, out of mind.

At the last minute, my conscience got the best of me, and I dragged myself to the patient's room to change her one last time. At least I was late leaving work for a better reason this time, and I'd be lying if I said I didn't have some small sense of pride that helped me ignore the pain in my feet and the ache in my bones.

Nursing is, for the most part, an autonomous occupation. Once you've got the credentials required for a particular scope of practice, as long as you can execute tasks within your knowledge, skill, and judgement, you can organize your shift the way you want. For better or worse, it's not an isolated job, and you are expected to work alongside teams of doctors, dieticians, physiotherapists, occupational therapists, social workers, and pharmacists. Despite the necessity to work as part of a team, living my personal life in comfortable isolation made me uncomfortable with this aspect of the job. I had difficulty asking for help in all parts of my life, and asking for it from colleagues was no different. I felt accountable for everything and tried to do it all on my own. As a child, I learned that caring was hard work, and taking a cue from my mom, my exhaustion signalled my level of commitment. The words of a particular charge nurse still haunt me to this day, as she once took me aside and forced me on a break after a stressful interaction with a patient.

"Don't worry about your patients, they aren't going to worry about you," she said.

I wish I could tell her how important it was for me to hear those words.

You often hear that a job is better when you work with people you like, but I never really cared to get close to my co-workers. I always had the mindset of getting the job done and going home. It seems having a sense of compassion in nursing is more of an asset than a requirement these days, and at the end of the day it was a job that provided a paycheck. The more my mind and body degraded, the more this became true. The gratitude I occasionally received from patients and family members paled in comparison to the amount of effort it required from me to complete the job, and the physical and emotional demands required of me. Eventually, the profession chipped away any resilience I had, and I was left to face the many years of my blatant self-neglect.

Although a desire to be acknowledged had always bubbled below the surface of my consciousness, moments in my life had validated the uselessness of my efforts to change. Staying shy and soft-spoken was an adaptation to the extroverts that would steamroll over me throughout my upbringing. I eventually became complacent to let my points go instead of dealing with the budding anger from multiple unsuccessful attempts to be heard. The effort was simply too draining for me. It was easier to live inside my mind alongside opinions that were never challenged or judged by those around me (even when part of it was due to cowardice). I was afraid to speak out, and I wore my silent suffering as some sort of badge of honour that entitled me to my misery.

I had always felt different than the people around me, which made me become bitter toward their happiness and my inability to find it. Envy has always been my deadliest sin.

Growing up surrounded by parental unease, moving homes, and my brother's oppressive moods, I adapted with the rationale of a turtle and drew myself inward. I was defensive—no one was allowed in this little world that I created in my head, and all I needed was myself. As anyone will tell you, the longer you try to suppress an uncomfortable emotion, the more likely it is to explode. The carefully cultivated silence of my childhood was no different, and the older I got, the more cynical I became. I was angry and harshly judged people who lived shamelessly with their emotions.

It's incredibly ironic that as someone who worked in a profession punctuated by compassion, I ignored my own needs. Despite the circumstances of my childhood preparing me for internal conflict, continuing to suppress my needs into adulthood disrupted my familiar quiet, reserved identity. A primal, anarchist scream bubbled like hot lava under the crust of my carefully constructed persona. I had isolated my mind, and my identity lived in a prison of my own creation. My soul was fighting for dominance over my body's need for survival, and I had to stretch the bonds of my vestigial desire for solitude somehow, or face complete inner chaos when I inevitably snapped.

I had to untangle myself from a past of staunchly conservative opinions as a coping mechanism, because I resented the infantile cynicism I had developed as a result. Although I feared the worst when it came to change and new experiences, a need to break free from the chains of the mundane drew me toward experiences on extreme ends of a spectrum where physical and metaphysical feelings merge. The first step was a shift in perspective, a willingness to be vulnerable and confront the parts of myself that I didn't like, and then to tell them kindly to chill the fuck out.

7
Leading Up

I needed something bigger than myself to believe in. Something big enough to take the focus off my inner turmoil, like my focus on others used to do. In this crisis of faith, I felt myself starting to succumb to an inner self that I could no longer ignore, but didn't know how yet to be. This isn't an isolated event in the history of humanity; with the evolution of our minds as a species came the painful intellect that needs to find a reason for everything. I was suffering, and there needed to be a reason for it.

Since I couldn't seem to dull the pain, I needed to find a reason for it. The only thing that made sense to me was to find a sense of purpose, or some predestined goal to work toward now that nursing had failed me. As a woman, society holds an expectation that our purpose is motherhood, which is supposed to fulfil us. I had no aspirations of having children, experiencing firsthand that parenthood was a life of hardship. Besides that, I knew the reason for this pain needed to be bigger than myself, and not just something to pass on to another generation. Reaching out for an answer, I wanted to find something reaching back for me and thirsty as I was for a distraction, I began to search.

I can't stand a waste of logic or intellect. The big, beautiful brains of our species have developed over centuries, and I firmly believe that the mind is a terrible thing to waste. Religion was created (I daresay even designed) to fulfil human need by placating our existential worries, but I felt that was too easy; to maintain that there is one supreme entity governing the universe, like the dominant religious belief in America, is in my humble opinion, incredibly ignorant. It can be tempting to believe in one reason, or being, behind every outcome which absolves us of all responsibility from our actions, but what's the point? Looking at all the infinite mysteries of the world we're still discovering to this day, there is simply so much we do not, and simply *cannot* know. At its worst, religion can punish and/or kill those with a difference of opinion, and at its best, it is an excuse for complacency.

I'm not an atheist. I'm a realist. Even call me a hopeless romantic.

For this reason, I separate spirituality from religion. Spirituality to me is an active belief: permitting oneself to explore options for living a meaningful life. The notion of spirituality allows the possibility for multiple "truths" that are different for each individual, exchanges a rigid nature in favour of gentle exploration, and is set in the background of a transcendental puzzle. Through spirituality, our beautiful minds can explore, seeking to overcome our biases toward others, and separate emotion from logic without sacrificing either.

I was inexperienced in both religious and spiritual practices. I never went to church, and I had never meditated, prayed, or even done yoga. I did, however, gravitate toward the occult, intrigued by the unknown and practices involving tarot cards, pendulums, numerology, palmistry, and astrology. As a millennial, I was part of the growing collective interest in these ancient predictive modalities, and to this day branches of science continue to analyze them. For example, psychology suggests that people who become obsessed with astrology and personality types are the children who were never understood at home; by trying to understand every nuance of another person, their unconscious desire is that someone would have done the same for them.

I was fixated on impossible knowledge and the secrets of the universe. If I explored realms of existence beyond what was visible with our eyes, I thought I could find an answer to what I was looking for.

For this reason, my path toward "Weedsdom" initially started out with psychedelic mushrooms.

I was always drawn to Native histories as the first cultures in a symbiotic relationship with the earth. Their oneness with the planet and their tales of communication with the spirit world naturally drew my interest. I admired the culture of early Indigenous Peoples and their practices of living off the resources of the land, as well as their respect of elders and the wisdom they bring to their communities. I thought this proposed a very natural order to life: living alongside the other creatures that share this planet with us, with everyone and everything having a role to play. Stories of the ceremonies and initiations used in their culture and the tales of visions fascinated me the most, offering a connection to another realm and the promise of transcendental knowledge. But how could we, as mere human beings, access this knowledge? Mother Nature seemed to hold the answer.

I figured it wouldn't be uncommon for psilocybin, also known as "magic" mushrooms (which contain psychedelic compounds causing hallucinogenic effects when ingested) to either accidentally or purposefully become the source of these visions. Naturally occurring in our environment, I could see how they may have been regarded as a gift from whatever gods existed. The historical use of cannabis also supports this, as it too was often used to invoke psychoactive, religious-like experiences throughout different cultures all over the world.

I wanted in on the knowledge, but I had no idea how to do it. The only thing I could think of was to consult my older brother Adam who, having evolved past the circumstances of his childhood, belly-flopped into the wonderful world of recreational drugs. Experienced with all the legal pharmaceuticals he was on as a child to control his Tourette's and behavioural issues, Adam performed an intellectual experiment to see what effects some of the more stigmatized ones had on the mind and body. He had always marched to the beat of his own drum—for better or for worse—and although I still had some small measure of fear toward him, I was also in awe of him. While I grew up being unable to ignore the voices in my head that scared me away from new experiences, he dived in head first, eager to make up for the moments without fear that he never got growing up.

I shocked him with my inquiry into how to procure and partake in magic "shrooms," but was blindsided instead when he advised me to first try weed. He suggested it would be less intense than the mushrooms to a novice such as myself, which was a thought later characterized by Jem's boyfriend Mike:

With weed: *"Oh, it's a spider."*
With mushrooms: *"Fuck! It's a spider!"*

I didn't know what to think, and I was torn between gratitude for the consideration of my sanity and the disappointment in being advised against my goal. Because of the association with spirituality, I never saw magic mushrooms as a drug, but rather as a tool. When it came to drugs, I immediately looked down on anyone who partook in such vices, harshly judging them as weak and pathetic in their inability to face life without chemical intervention (ironic since I had been on antidepressant medication since my childhood). I prided myself on having never smoked or done anything harsher than the occasional alcoholic beverage to loosen up. Alcohol was always celebrated and never included in the forbidden substance line-up (Stay tuned, I have a tirade on that later).

I defended these strong views to myself to justify my voluntary isolation from society, although I suppose one benefit of being an introvert is that peer pressure is not as much of an issue. Unconsciously influenced by society's stern rules (drugs are bad mmmmkay?), my harsh opinions were able to thrive on my lack of association with users, or from the influence of others in general.

I had never even considered an indulgence in cannabis, having been turned off to smoking from years of my mother's cigarette habit. I was ignorant, and it didn't help that the images fed to me from society were that of dreadlocks, slow movement, and general uselessness clouded by a haze of reefer smoke. As a (mostly) reformed snob, I appeal to you to think on what you read, as I feel it both as a duty and a personal necessity to share my experiences. Should they result in your own introspection, or simply your amusement, that is your prerogative. My intention is not to encourage the consumption of cannabis to those opposed. My hope is to address its stigma throughout time, pointing out the stupidity behind society's narrative that allows the legal consumption of deadlier substances. At the very least, I hope to entertain you with stories of my personal discoveries and follies, and to present a different depiction than the traditional pot-head or stoner.

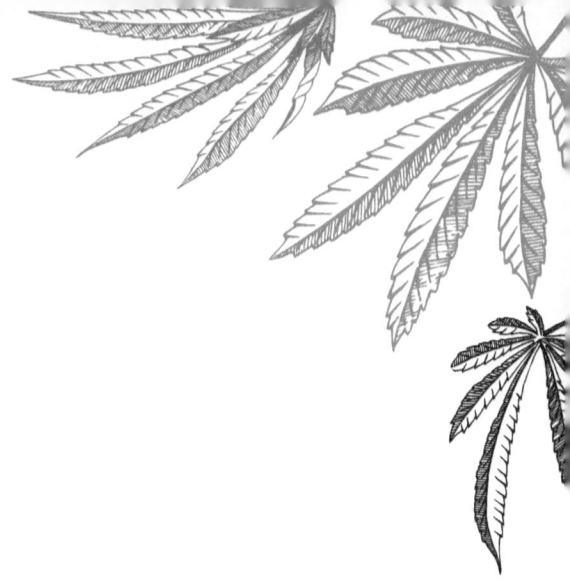

PART II:
IN GOOD
COMPANY

8
My First Deal

I always relied on Adam and Jem to interact with (what I considered) the underworld of society on my behalf. They were my access to those I imagined on the dirty side of my illicit drug habit: the people who always knew how to get the good stuff if you wanted to take a walk on the wild side. It wasn't that I thought I was better than either of them, I was really just a coward. I was intimidated by anyone who didn't succumb to their fears like I usually did, and I was afraid to get caught; cannabis wasn't legal back then as it is now. When the joints Adam gave me were long gone and I felt like I was getting on Jem's nerves by always relying on her supply, I decided it was time to act like an adult and get my own drugs. Not knowing where to start, I once again reached out for Adam's support. After all, what's family for?

Of course, my brother knew a guy. He assured me "his stuff is solid," and I pretended to understand what that meant. I felt like a narc, which made me feel more nervous about the whole thing. I texted the number Adam gave me, dropping his name into the message like a password to establish my innocence. The guy on the other end seemed friendly and non-intimidating, although it was like pulling teeth trying to steer the conversation without spelling out my needs completely. It turned out he was a travelling salesman, and he agreed to come to me at my apartment. Although it was during the daytime, and Adam had vouched for him, fear spread from my mind and tingled at the back of my neck as I considered my safety. And yet, I knew I was ready.

When my phone rang to signal a visitor at the front entrance of my building, I buzzed him in and spent the time waiting for him to arrive at my door by pacing back and forth and wringing my hands. It wasn't long before the knock came, and I opened it to see a young, handsome, shaggy-haired kid. He carried a beige saddle-bag over his shoulder and extended his hand to me in greeting. I found it hard not to focus on his right arm, which was covered in a tattoo sleeve of indistinct patterns visible to his elbow. His politeness was an unexpected pleasure, and as we shook hands, he asked to come inside.

He removed his shoes—holey Converse sneakers with dirty shoe-laces—by the door and requested to sit. I forced out my arm, clumsily extending my twenty dollar bill at him.

"Oh! Thank you very much," he said, and sat down on the chair in front of my cheap dining room table, dropping the money on top. I was reminded how embarrassingly out of my element I was.

Aren't drug deals supposed to be quick? You hand someone the money, they hand you the product . . . generally in some clandestine slight-of-the-hand. Giving payment first is a sign of good faith, right? Isn't it? Like ladies of the night you've got to get paid up front. Don't you?

Nope. Not in this case at least—I got some world-class customer service.

Sitting at the table, Boy-o pulled out a big Bick's pickle jar FULL of beautiful nuggets of weed.

"What kind do you want?" he asked me as I stood there, dumbfounded.

Mmmmmm, pickles.

"Uhh, the smoking variety?" I eventually said.

I couldn't even hazard a guess at what he had in stock, and edibles were far too ambitious for me at this point, so I didn't bother to ask.

Thankfully, my idiocy was met with acceptance and he nodded softly, unscrewing the lid of his pickle jar.

"Can I weigh it for you?" he asked, reaching down once again into the beige saddlebag at his feet. I shrugged, fairly sure that it was a rhetorical question. I would have rather reached into the jar and pulled out a handful of those magnificent nuggets shouting "this many!" in childish glee, but thankfully, I managed to compose myself.

He pulled out a small, flat, black device from his bag—an imagined cornucopia to my hungry eyes—and placed the scale onto the table. Gently reaching into the pickle jar, he cupped each nugget in his forefingers, and pulled out one out at a time, placing each on the scale. Digital numbers appeared on the small screen, which measured out the transaction with clinical accuracy, and he added to it until it hit a rounded sum of two grams for twenty bucks. Gathering my purchase, he sealed it in an adorably tiny plastic bag. Pulling out another small bag, he paired it with my purchase.

"This is White Viper," he said, holding my initial product. "And this is Orange Kush" motioning to the unexpected addition. "I'll give you some of this to try, and you can get it next time if you like it."

With the transaction complete, I thanked him, took my tiny packages, and walked him to the door of my apartment to put his shoes back on. Swinging his bag over his shoulder, he extended a hand once again.

"Very nice to meet you," he said and smiled, showing a set of straight, white teeth, and as I took his hand I couldn't help but return a smile of my own. He turned and headed down the hallway toward the floor's elevators, and I closed the door softly behind him. Turning to look out my balcony window, the sun was shining brightly through the glass, inviting me to come out and play. My excitement spiked as I mentally crafted my review, as any good consumer would do to favour a small business:

Pleasant young gentleman with professional level of customer service who knows his stuff. Polite and courteous. A pleasure to do business with. Five stars. Would highly recommend.

9
Kitkat

As a solitary creature and introvert, I was always more content to sit on the sidelines watching and learning what went on around me. I preferred to listen to a conversation rather than lead one, and being around others and talking at length would often tire me out. It was a vicious cycle, because supressing my own desires and needs also meant I was dependant on limited interaction with other people. Even though I had friends, I had very few that I actually opened up to by sharing the lonely history of my childhood, or expressing my innermost thoughts and dreams. I much preferred the company of animals. With animals, there is no pretense—we know we are different creatures. This is why I resonated more with the pets I kept company with, particularly my cats.

There is a general belief that cats are assholes, always clawing at your furniture and puking on your belongings as they claim their territory and spread their scent of possession. I think this dignified nature was always a part of the species, but after their domestication they became smaller, and some people become uneasy with pretentious personalities in small packages. Cats are very different from dogs, which will follow you to the ends of the earth with their loyalty, and they tend to act—for the most part—like they couldn't give a shit about where you go or what you do as long as you feed them. To a dog, you are their best friend and companion. To a cat, you are *their* pet, and a nuisance to be tolerated at best. One of the best quotes I've ever heard was from author Terry Pratchett, who said, "In ancient times cats were worshiped as gods; they have not forgotten this."

I've always personally preferred cats over dogs; I relate to the comfort they have in their independence. It's been suggested that people who don't like cats have a problem with boundaries. Because cats are very clear when your actions make them uncomfortable (they will bite, hiss, or scratch), you have to develop a relationship with them at their speed. For some reason, just because they're considered pets, some people feel this entitles them to demand what they want from cats, and then not like it when there are repercussions to their actions.

I developed close bonds with a few special cats throughout my life, and I like to think they had a soft spot in their furry hearts for me too. My dad has a picture of me as a child sitting on the couch of our first family home with Kiddo 2, who was a grey and white striped tabby named after his predecessor, Kiddo 1 (both were named by my dad using his literal sense of humour). In the picture, Kiddo 2 is curling a paw over my knee, both of us rapt in attention to the television in front of us.

I grew up with my first cat, an overweight orange tabby named Pal, who had an effeminate nature. He tended to mother everyone and everything by climbing up beside you, placing a paw over your leg, and imploring you to pat him with his gentle smile before he licked you relentlessly with his sandpaper tongue. He was a friendly giant who would knead you like a kitten, purr uncontrollably, and gaze at you lovingly—in genuine appreciation of your company—as he sat with you. Even my grandmother, who was generally stoic in nature, couldn't resist his charm and surrendered to his whims with a few pats on his head. When he was suffering from old age, we hoped he would die peacefully at home so we could have him with us for as long as possible, but the time came when he could no longer lay without struggling to breathe. Watching him on his favourite spot on the living room couch, he crouched restlessly, wheezing in short, frequent bursts that tore at my heart strings. I told my mom we had to take him to the vet, knowing full well we wouldn't be coming home with him. As any pet lover will tell you, putting down a pet is losing a member of your family, and it's nothing short of heart-wrenching.

As close as I was to Pal growing up, a new relationship awaited me that would bring me a different, deeper form of love. I was much older by then, in my early twenties and ready to embark on a new stage of adulthood that started with my career in nursing and living on my own. Having grown up with animals around me all my life, I was loathe to stop. I wanted a companion that could be comfortable enough at home on their own while I was doing my shift work, but that wasn't confined to a cage or tank. Fish were out, as I proved to be a poor caretaker in the past. I neglected to clean the tank after their novelty wore out, and I discovered their inability to hold eye contact. My dad was the one who took pity on my fish when he dropped me off at Mom's, staying to wipe the grime off the glass as he scolded me for my indifference to their fate. We both sighed in relief when they flushed successfully down the toilet to their watery graves, bloated as they were from my tendency to displace my guilt by overfeeding them.

I had also dabbled in the small and fuzzy. Hamsters, although cute, give even *less* of a shit about you than cats, hide during the day, and spiral incessantly at night on their wheels. Rats were always out because of parental discrimination—apparently their tails resemble snakes too much. My last rodent was a guinea pig named Taffy, who, much to my dismay, would only snuggle up next to me when she wanted to pee, chirping deviously before she did. Rabbits were soft but soulless, and their smell-to-cuddling ratio was even narrower than Taffy's. Nope. I was done with creatures that walked and pooped simultaneously. As much as I love dogs, they were far too needy, and I still had to learn to take care of myself. Another cat seemed like the best choice in terms of temperament, self-sufficiency, and positive past experiences. I decided I wanted to adopt, and this was how I came to own the third denizen of the bachelorette pad Jem and I inhabited.

An older cat with an unusual name, Kitkat had history. Previously named Katka, she had been adopted as a kitten and returned to the shelter when she was seven. Having a history of abandonment, she was justifiably on edge when the shelter staff opened her cage to stick their hand in, effectively cornering her to introduce us. Even though this made her seem unfriendly, I saw potential. When I showed interest in her, the staff were ecstatic because they were starting to lose hope that she would be adopted. Although a proclaimed sweetheart, Katka was a returned product: elderly and all black, which meant she was less likely to be adopted again due to superstition (because apparently that's still a thing).

I was guided to a small room with floor-length glass windows and a couple of chairs, where families went to "interview" their adoptees. Kitkat was plopped down on the floor before me as I entered, and the staff member smiled, gave a thumbs-up, and closed the door softly behind us. While Kitkat started sniffing and smearing her scent on everything without so much as a backwards glance at me, I began to plan for our future. I hated the name Katka, and I wanted to change the shelter name in the same symbolic way an emancipated slave regains their freedom. Because she was older, I figured she might be too stubborn to respond to change, but I began to list all the names I could think of that had a hard 'K,' which would be similar enough.

In a flash it came to me, and like calling the name of a sadistic ghoul from the eighties, I proudly released her new name from my lips. Whether it was because my voice had just reminded her of my presence, or the linguistics were indeed familiar to her, she stopped and turned her head to make eye contact with me. She had me at "Mrrow."

The rest fell into place easily; I left the meeting room to tell the staff of my decision, and picked her up the next day. She was with me before I moved in with Jem, and although she was physically small, Kitkat was as big a personality as either of us, claiming her role as an additional roommate. As much as she tried to act indifferent and pretend my existence was merely to be tolerated, I knew she loved me, and I knew she knew that I knew.

Although less complex than with a human soul, I developed a close personal relationship with my cat and—scoff if you will—I found that when I was under the influence of weed, it was easier to understand her. When her voice rang out in her characteristic wheezy chirp, I naturally translated her dialect to that of an elderly matron, large and in charge. I imagined her as a model or dancer in a previous life, retaining her youthful beauty even as her body aged traitorously. A survivor like Scarlett O'Hara in *Gone with the Wind*, she remembered the good life, and damned if she would settle for anything less.

Jem judged her fairly as "aesthetically pleasing" with a classic profile (for a cat), round face, and big green eyes that contrasted nicely with the ebony gloss of her fur. Kitkat was a bossy little thing, unafraid to seek me out if I failed her expectations, and often came after me when I fed her without the usual zest of my rampant affections by singing or praising her beauty.

"What the fuck?! You did it wrong!" I often translated.

While I was high, she'd lead me, as if on autopilot, back to the kitchen, squawking the whole way with her hips flaring, looking over her shoulder to see that I was still following. I would look down at her food dish to see that the pâté I unceremoniously plopped down in her dish had been licked dry, and because she was old and spoiled, she couldn't be bothered to bite into its solid form, preferring instead to have me take the work out of it by mashing it up with a fork.

I took great delight in examining the nature of cats, especially in realizing how their territorial nature manifested as two main behaviours: Cleanse (lick) and smear (rub scent on things). Having scent glands practically everywhere on their bodies (including the sides of their face), rubbing themselves on things is how they mark what they own. Some of the typically more annoying traits were an endless source of amusement for me, like the subtle power-flex Kitkat exercised when she walked ahead of me and stopped as I was mid-stride, spreading out to halt my progress and pay attention to her. Or the times she would burst through my bedroom door, irate and squawking, when I kept it closed in the winter to keep the warmth of my heater circulating. I translated:

"I just saw you go in there, but are you in there?! How dare you shut me out!"

10
Jem

I've been best friends with Jem since we were both in daycare, long before we became roommates. I started at a new school when I entered grade two, and after classes she and I connected through our mutual love of Barbie dolls, Disney, Sailor Moon, and beef-flavoured ramen noodles while we waited for our moms (both single parents) to take us home. The adventurous platinum-haired child became my closest friend throughout childhood, and when I was in a receptive mood, we spent most of our time together obsessing over more of the same things. When we went to different high schools, we fell out of each other's lives, but every so often, one of us would reach out to connect once again. Like any true friendship, despite the amount of time that's passed, it's always easy to pick up where you left off like nothing has changed. She was a great support when I discovered cannabis, and was perhaps even part of its inception since she was no stranger to it.

Jem has a soul that lights up every room with its aura, and the lights around me often seem to glow brighter when she comes into a room. Her eyes are the soft colour of a sapphire, and when she laughs they sparkle faintly. Only when I look at her directly, behind the dainty hand she holds in front of her face like the fan of a Japanese geisha, can I see her eyes tightly shut when she finds something really funny.

She has an innocence I've often compared to Meeko, the raccoon from the Disney version of *Pocahontas*. She has a fearless sense of curiosity, a wide, tight-lipped smile, and a childish excitement for food that causes her to smack her lips in anticipation. She is the Benicio Del Toro to my Johnny Depp (as in *Fear and Loathing in Las Vegas),* when she advises me like an attorney with her silver tongue, casually lighting up a bong.

Although we had always talked about living together when we were young, when we actually started to as adults in our mid-twenties, I think there was always unspoken fear because of our different natures. Our family situations were similar, but there were a few key differences too.

Jem was an only child (until much later in her life) while I grew up with an older brother, and her dad wasn't involved in her upbringing while mine was, despite how minimal a role he seemed to have. I was more of a loner who would rather stay inside and play a video game than go out and socialize, while Jem was more outgoing and personable. She was more physically involved in activities, while I detested the thought of sports. Her music taste leaned toward the hardcore, like rock and rap, while I preferred pop or the oldies from its association with my dad. I focused on the domestic doll life when we played together with our Barbies, intent on falling in love with my favourite Ken doll. While I indulged as a young romantic, playing out the epic romances of my imagination, Jem played on the move by emulating parties, grand adventures with multiple wardrobe changes, and riding on horseback through the perilous mountains of furniture. Annoyed by her inability to stay still, I sat grumbling next to my carefully-constructed fort of pillow cushions, wishing she would bring her entourage to visit my picture-perfect family.

Despite our opposite natures, the most important thing that helped our friendship stand the test of time was our history together. As children, Jem and I lived down the street from each other, on the opposite sides of a wide bridge that crossed one of the main highways of the city. In the summer months we took turns crossing against the busy hum of traffic below on our way to each other's houses. We often spent our days together riding our bikes down residential streets to explore the nearby construction sites of the booming housing developments. Surrounded by the skeletons of homes and dirt hills, we created our adventures, making up stories about what superpowers we would want to have, how we would look, and the love triangles we would get ourselves into.

On the playground outside my childhood home, we jumped fearlessly off the top level of a rectangular wooden structure for the sake of drama. Laughter would quickly break the tension. Jem once laid on the coarse sand below, draped her arm dramatically across her forehead, and stated, "Pretend I'm dead," just as the wind passed by to blow her dress up over her head, panties exposed to all.

Light-hearted encounters also had a tendency to turn tense, like the time Jem found a set of ancient lawn darts in her garage that she brought with us to the top of our favourite dirt hill in the construction area across from her house. Brightly coloured and roughly the size of our childish forearms, we discovered later (much to my amusement) that these darts were recalled for safety reasons. Something to do with their sharp metal tips.

We climbed to the top of the hill and, after finding a flat patch of grass, Jem tossed one of the bright-yellow missiles into the sky. I barely registered her movement, as I was distracted by the surprising amount of greenery at the peak, and anxious about the thistles scratching my exposed flesh—it would itch like a bitch later.

I suspect the situation was similar to a shark attack: if you were swimming and minding your own business, you might become disoriented by the speed and force of some obnoxious object pushing you away from your centre of balance. Looking down, you may be thankful for the way your body absorbs the shock of seeing a stream of blood pooling around you. I didn't hear anything before I was struck from above by the dart, and I only felt the force of a blunt object hit my head. I'd been hit in the head many times before—once face-first by a rogue dodge ball during recess in public school; my brief life had flashed before my eyes, while a faint "sorry" whispered from the background of my repose.

I reached my hand to touch the impact point, and looked down at the smear of bright red on my fingers. The gash on my head from the aerial mini-spear wasn't too deep, and thankfully all my limbs were still intact after the attack. Due to my shock, I barely felt anything, but there was a look of calm hurry on Jem's face (explained as sheer terror to me years later) as we rushed back to her house to cover up the bloody evidence before we got in trouble. (There was no need to tell the adults– *clearly* I'm fine now!)

Given her rather tumultuous family life, Jem ended up following the path of her dolls, moving far from home and into the bowels of the city, far earlier than my eventual venture out of the suburbs. We talked less frequently and eventually drifted apart from the physical divide between us. Once we reconnected in the city as young adults, it was relieving to discover that we were able to pick up (more or less), where we left off.

Over a bowl of our favourite beef-flavoured noodles, we revisited the idea of living together as besties. My lease was ending with my current roommates, and she was looking to escape hers. Like an old box from the attic that gets dusted off, circumstances were finally right to put our plan into motion. Despite the years that had passed between us and the experiences we never got to share, we found each other again, and it felt like the natural order of things to be together.

The shared history between us made it easy to reconnect, and with Jem by my side during my foray into drugs, my psychoactive journey was enhanced by my comfort level. Whether we were having deeply profound conversations wondering about the morality of humanity, or typical stoner thoughts like casually discussing the merits of buying and owning a deep fryer, we never felt judged by each other. We were a kind of comfortable where you could shamelessly admit mid-conversation that you had no idea what you were just talking about. With Jem, the friendship we already shared was magnified, and we often reflected on shared experiences under one influence.

11

Porch Ladies

Inspired by our leisurely gathering outdoors to partake in cannabis, Jem and I created an identity for ourselves as "Porch Ladies" (or synonymously, "Balcony Broads"). Our porch was our balcony on the nineteenth floor of an apartment building, and it was nothing short of a passageway to discovery in our heightened minds when Jem and I smoked. The complex we lived in was one of two tucked behind a row of houses on a popular strip of Toronto's "Greektown." The buildings faced each other, making the balconies of each apartment face their neighbours across. Stacked on top of each other, the balconies looked like little backyards. It made ours seem more like a porch from where we could sit and look out at the lives of our neighbours without intending to be creepy about it.

Our view offered the vastness of the sky and the expanse of the busy city underneath us. In the middle of a thunderstorm, we watched from our shelter outside, shielded by the concrete surroundings of our balcony and the one above us. Rain pelted sideways into the trees below, and omnipotent gusts of wind stretched their branches back from the directions they grew toward. After the storm's passing, we marvelled at the rainbow stretching far and wide along the city line and contemplated how the ashes of a cigarette from a neighbour above floated down to us, flickering like burning rain.

In the summer, Jem would perch her Blackberry phone inside of one of our kitchen bowls to amplify the sound of the music we played (she was always coming up with ingeniously simple solutions to our first-world problems). Since our balcony overlooked a busy city highway, it was always very loud during the day, but Jem's modern survival skills always kept us going. When the days were especially warm, we left the balcony door open and Kitkat would occasionally venture out with us, prowling around cautiously for just long enough to make me nervous of her exploring the edge too intimately and falling. It was enclosed well, but with the paranoia of the weed in full swing, I became a mother hen clucking at my adventurous child. If she wasn't outside, she was inside contemplating the outside, only to want inside again. And then deciding she wanted outside.

It wouldn't matter to us when winter came to the city, because the Porch Ladies were never discouraged to go outside and partake in our herb of choice; we would simply prepare using a checklist.

Blankets? *Check.*
Earmuffs? *Check.*
Boots? *Check.*
Single glove à la Michael Jackson style? (For the hand holding the joint that was exposed to the cold) *Check.*
Pyjamas? (Comfort over beauty) *Check.*

Like little old ladies we bundled up in our layers and prepared for the elements, enduring the cold in our accoutrements, plus or minus an alcoholic indulgence on the weekends. We lit up our bong and puffed like chimneys to herald the resiliency of Canadians surviving in the winter; there was life within this arctic climate, and it didn't die easily.

While the residents around us probably believed, like we did, that we maintained our privacy beyond the glass doors of our balcony, we soon realized that this wasn't always true. On one occasion we were able to see an entire living room and its occupants, circled around the focal point—a large flat-screen TV—watching some movie with subtitles, and eating some unknown nourishment from the bowls they hunched over. The vulnerability of realizing that our lives must be similarly reflected to others was thankfully dulled under the haze of a high, and Jem and I came to laugh at how we must appear to anyone who happened to be watching.

Our preoccupations included wiggling our arm fat in the breeze, shaking our arms back and forth like chickens, or sitting with our jaws slack and mouths open, trying (in our inebriated minds) to relax the muscles in our faces. We occasionally lit candles during the night, partaking in the occult by attempting to cast spells and enchantments (Jem had more a flair for this than I did). It was always a fun practice to guess what our neighbours could be saying if they happened to look out their window at us, and I liked to imagine the conversation as they yelled to their husband/wife/partner/roommate:

"Harold! Come 'ere and look at what those crazy idiots are doing over there now! They got a candle or some shit!"

Of course, Harold would come, shuffling through the hallway over to the window and join in.

"Christ! They doin' witchcraft now?! Dumb fuckers must be on drugs."

We must have looked like the dumbest shits, but this is a crux of the marijuana issue: although assuredly looking like an idiot to the general public, I can tell you in utmost confidence we were having our minds blown by the simplicities of living in the present moment.

Jem did practice witchcraft, but only the practical kind, and it often came in handy. The first (and only) time I went to a fetish club, I was "bitten" by a vampire: A French gentleman from Montreal named Jerome. He had custom implants on his canine teeth that gave him the fangs of a vampire, and boy did he leave one hell of a hickey (it was surprisingly even in diameter around my neck . . . damn those sexy French). Note to the wise, don't agree to go to a fetish club the night before work if you don't want to get teased or judged mercilessly.

Luckily, Jem had been taking a Holistic Health Practitioner program at the time, and divulged excitedly,

"Oh! I have an aromatic oil for drawing out blood and speeding healing!"

As she began to mix lotions and oils together with her pinky finger, all I could think of was:

Witch! Mixing a potion!

Thank goodness Mr. Potter made magic cool again, because the knowledge is just as old as the superstition. Earlier, when I sensed I was catching a cold, Jem concocted a mixture of eucalyptus and tea tree oil to put near the shower and told me the heat would activate the antibacterial properties of the oil to fight my cold.

When Jem gave me the hickey tincture, she said,

"Just be warned the blood will come to the surface, and it'll look really nasty for a while."

I learned not to question the craft. Any good witch will tell you it's all about intention.

Unfortunately herbomancy (the use of flora, fungi, trees, and the like for magical purposes), was neither of our strong suits when it came to the practice of witchcraft. Although we desired house plants, our record for the consistent nurturing of them was very poor. The few survivors we had were all Jem's, but even they lingered perilously close to certain demise. I had a small basil plant which was pre-packaged to grow (and had like, three instructions), and I still managed to kill it by either forgetting about it or over-watering it in the same fashion an overbearing, but well-meaning, parent may smother their child.

One summer, we decided that those pre-potted plants from the grocery store were a safe bet against our propensity for negligence, and propped several lovingly on our balcony. Tending to our new recruits was a magical experience under the influence of a high. The small, fuzzy leaves of our oregano and lavender plants were as soft as puppies.

With my acquired tunnel vision, I felt like I could see the embryology behind their growth: the buds of the leaves sprouting from the genetic material, which was carried up through the stems, all originated from a small, single seed. I stroked and parted each tiny structure, feeling the earthly connection to its components and how it was alive yet separate in consciousness from us as humans. Free from the burden of choice, it existed on earth to survive with the singular purpose of propagation, but without the weight of disappointment if it should not succeed in that purpose. This contrasted starkly with the inevitable disappointment Jem and I both felt when all our plants died yet again.

The only plant that managed to stay alive in the apartment was a small tree that Jem kept with her over the years she lived on her own in the city. The small, gnarled root remained in its oversized white pot, buried by a small layer of dry dirt. Lovingly referred to as the "elephant tree," its bark resembled the lined and weathered skin of the creature, and its little stubby branches made it look similar to their feet. I don't know what type of plant it actually was, but no matter how long it was before Jem remembered to water it, it seemed to stay in relatively good health, occasionally sprouting some leaves or growing longer branches. We ruminated on the immortality of the elephant tree: could we ingest and digest this tree and live forever?

Just asking the real questions . . .

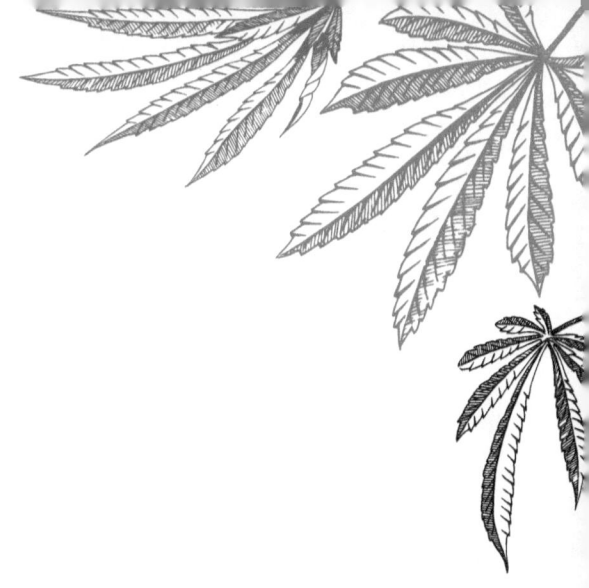

PART III: KNOW THINE ENEMY

12
(Modern) History

It's pretty easy to learn how different cultures have used (and continue to use) psychoactive drugs for medicine, religion, recreation, or rebellion. Given the information-age of technology we live in, almost anything is accessible. While this is generally beneficial, every light can cast a shadow, and misinformation and bias threatens every search. Trailblazers throughout the existence of humanity have pursued knowledge by challenging these shadows, and thankfully, as society progresses, there are more of us who question previously established societal norms.

For example, centuries ago you could face death if one of your neighbours ratted you out for collecting herbs in your garden. *(Witchcraft! Unholy knowledge of the devil!)* These days, you can now walk proudly into a bookstore and pick up a copy of the popular *Necronomicon*, H.P Lovecraft's fictional grimoire commonly known as the "Book of the Dead," alongside "A Beginner's Guide to Aromatherapy" marked down at fifty percent off its original price.

Yes sir, the times are a-changing! When it comes to modern society and our norms, I like to think we're moving in the right direction when we consider the things that were once taboo. However, certain things have frustratingly stayed the same, like views on drugs. Heck, even the word "drugs" can invoke a visceral response in most people, and one that is historically planted. Even now, governments play "Mama knows best" by picking and choosing which substances should be taboo and which are acceptable. Make no mistake, there are reasons behind which are chosen, which aren't, and why. Most of the time, you'll find the answer by following the reciprocal relationship between who (or what) holds the money and the power.

There has been a war on drugs in America since the beginning of the country's founding, and it's well documented. It is particularly used to alienate minorities, creating a narrative of "Us" versus "Them." *We* don't do drugs. *We* aren't losers like *they* are. *We* are better than *them*. After all, isn't that unconsciously imbued in nationalism?

Cannabis was once referred to as "The Devil's Lettuce" by Senior Douchebag Harry J. Ainslinger, who was the first head of the Federal Bureau of Narcotics in 1930, and let me tell you, this guy was a real piece of work. Ainslinger used the Spanish term for marijuana, "marihuana," as a weapon to justify racism against Mexican Americans and other minorities. He blamed the corruption of the drug for crimes committed by minorities, and preached to the masses about how smoking a joint would turn you into a psychopath who would murder your entire family. You would think this guy was sexually molested by (with?) a joint as a child, the way he attacked the issue with the vehemence of a personal vendetta, although according to Johann Hari, author of *Chasing the Scream: The First and Last Days of the War on Drugs*, Ainslinger was just crazy-racist, and scared of addicts.

In 1937, he continued his warpath with the *Marihuana Tax Act* that was passed by Congress in the United States, imposing a special tax on the substance. Although cannabis wasn't quite illegal, this was the beginning of imposing strict regulations on its distribution and use. The guy had no shame, and even targeted jazz musicians (because, you know, they were black) offended by their music and the growing cry against racism.

The first real contester to Ainslinger's Marihuana march-of-terror was New York mayor Fiorello La Guardia, who in 1944 reported findings from a panel of scientific sources opposing Ainslinger's fear mongering "facts" about cannabis. The La Guardia Committee, as the report is commonly referred to, proved that marijuana was not addicting "in the medical sense of the word," and that the association between marijuana creating criminals and delinquents was unfounded. Despite the five years of research that was presented by professionals in this report, Ainslinger denounced it as "unscientific" and little changed. He was a strong voice as the United States representative in the Single Convention on Narcotic Drugs of 1961, which was a meeting of the United Nations meant to establish, control, and enforce drug laws. In the US, this meeting helped established the Drug Enforcement Administration's Controlled Substances Act, and effectively lumped cannabis into Schedule I status, with the highest level of potential for abuse and severe psychological and/or physical dependence (Thanks a lot, Ass-Linger).

Despite repeated proposals to re-classify cannabis because of its well-documented medicinal benefits, it continues to be classified as a Schedule I substance. The US is slowly making progress, and we have come a long way from those douchebag-Ainslinger times. As of 2022, although cannabis is still illegal on a federal scale, most states allow for its medical use as long as it's prescribed by a physician, and a growing number of states have decriminalized or legalized it for adult recreational use. The rest of the world seems to be just as divided in terms of recreational legalisation and the levels of sentencing that come with one's association with the drug. Slowly, the collective consciousness of our world is shifting from its old ways, but our history is nuanced, and humanity is wary when it comes to change.

In 2019, Canada made cannabis legal for recreational use, but since we are (for better or for worse) heavily influenced by our obese neighbour to the south, it's important to know the history. While I was in my local library learning some of it, I was guided to the reference section of children's nonfiction, to a book series called *Incredibly Disgusting Drugs* published in 2008. I guess it makes sense to find such relics in a public house of knowledge.

The incredibly aggressive (and often offensive) approach of the volume covering marijuana scolded me like a child from each page, and in such a ridiculous fashion that it bordered on the exaggerated tales told around a campfire:

"By trying pot, even just once, you could be on the road to becoming a drug addict."

"People who use marijuana are known as potheads, dopeheads, druggies, burnouts, stoners, or just losers."

"Using pot . . . means you will never become a mature person who is worthy of respect from others."

I couldn't help but laugh, gasp, and angrily shake my head at the demeaning tone of the book, and I was disgusted to find this outdated piece of propaganda (perpetuating an Ainslinger-type legacy built on fear tactics) in a public library. This patronizing approach to educating children made me shudder to think of the generations to come, growing up with a deeply engrained sense of guilt for their natural adolescent curiosity and desire to explore the world around them. Then again, my mom always said her generation was raised on guilt.

I find it incredibly ironic that countries seem to acknowledge that children are the future, place responsibility on their upbringing to create a more inclusive society, and yet choose to groom them with such blatant fear tactics. It was certainly Ainslinger's tactic to divide the world, and it's a slippery slope when we become cruel to those that have the audacity to think differently.

Historical evidence suggests that the use of drugs started out with good intentions. Medical doctors were (and usually are) the first to experiment with substances with the most noble intent. For instance, did you know that ecstasy or MDMA (a psychedelic stimulant) was once used in psychotherapy and counseling? Psychiatrist George Greer, and his wife Requa Tolbert, a psychiatric nurse, conducted research with MDMA and low doses of ketamine in the 1980s before it was made illegal. In his testimony addressing the DEA on its place in the Controlled Substance Act, Greer stated that the drug's unique action was "a cutting through of the neurophysiological mechanisms of fear." In this altered state of consciousness, he noted improved communication and introspection from his patients, and that they were able to "communicate normally repressed ideas, memories, beliefs, opinions, and attitudes about themselves and others."

Some of the most notable historical figures and artists are known to have dabbled in both illicit and legal substances. Sigmund Freud, one of the most notable psychoanalysts of the twentieth century, was known to use cocaine. Aldous Huxley, well-known English writer of the chilling dystopian novel *Brave New World*, was a fan of alcohol, LSD, and mescaline. Hell, even Alexander the Great was reportedly drunk most of the time according to historians, and the guy is a literal legend. In his satirical poem, *Don Juan*, Lord Byron (a British poet of the early nineteenth century) wrote, "Man, being reasonable, must get drunk; the best of life is but intoxication." According to Marcus Aurelius (Roman Emperor, allegedly stoned on opium most of the time) in his *Meditations volume VIII*, "the denial of emotions is the key to transcending the troubles and pains of the material world . . . if thou art pained by any external thing, it is not this that disturbs thee, but thy own judgement about it. And it is in thy power to wipe out this judgement now." In other words, it's our judgements about things that hurt us rather than these things themselves, and by understanding our emotions we are put in a position of control to transcend any pain they may cause us. Tell me these aren't some original Words of Weedsdom.

Such profound thoughts have come from the minds of these respected figures of the past, who are known to have been under the influence of various substances. It's even been suggested that some (maybe most) of these figures were full-blown addicts. It stands to reason that addiction is not just a contagion of weak-willed burnouts, lowlifes, and losers that misguided children's books would have us believe.

13
Drugs

Let's talk about some of the legal drugs in America. In the words of William S. Burroughs, American author of the drug-fuelled novel *Naked Lunch:* "Our national drug is alcohol. We tend to regard the use of any other drug with special horror." Of course, America is nothing if not opportunistic, and if history is any indication, our views fluctuate in ways that benefit us. One could even argue that legal substances are regulated because society has collectively agreed that although we know they're bad for us, we don't want to live without them. Remember the Prohibition Era? That didn't work out so well, did it?

The discovery of alcohol as an intoxicant can be traced back to ancient Egypt and China around 7000 B.C. where it was thought to pay an important role in religion, medicine, and "social cohesion" by enhancing the quality and pleasures of life. Ironically, it's responsible for about 3 million deaths per year globally, which is more than any other substance, according to the World Health Organization (WHO). It's been scientifically proven that alcohol intoxication can cause irreversible organ damage or death, and that absorbing high concentrations can affect the brain's ability to control breathing, causing someone to pass out. Even while passed out, our bodies can continue to absorb alcohol, causing blood levels to reach dangerous levels that can kill us while we sleep—if we don't suffocate on our own vomit first, that is.

It's also common knowledge that alcohol intoxication doesn't just affect the user but can cause a danger to others as well; it's often a common denominator in violent crimes and domestic abuse. It has permeated into our culture so much that alcohol-related sponsorships of sporting and cultural events are common. Beer companies often sponsor boxing and other combat sports, creating an uncomfortable resonance with alcohol's role in promoting violence. Its presence is long-standing in our society, and its dangerous and debilitating effects have been observed, documented, and condemned throughout the ages. Governments try to impose regulations on alcohol consumption through age limits, but as you may know personally from your youth (as I do from mine), demand will always be met with supply, and adolescents are able to quite easily get their hands on it.

Age restrictions aside, many dangerous substances remain legal and accessible. We are free to pick our poison, and are even encouraged to do so by advertisements, as long as they absolve themselves with a warning like "please drink responsibly." Discreet boxes of text are easily slapped on a can of a popular energy drink to mention how it can negatively affect the heart. Warning labels on cigarette packages use all sorts of nasty pictures (tried-and-true fear tactics) to dissuade smokers. Even the paper inserts slipped inside your prescription drug packets listing all the possible side effects are legal protection for companies. All these substances remain legal as long as there is informed consent, and the companies wipe their hands clean of the consequences with federal blessings and an "at least we warned them."

I'm not saying alcohol should be banned (we all know that didn't work anyway), and I've had my fair share of indulgence as an adult. I'm just pointing out the hypocrisy of society and its judgements. Through the years we've learned more about the detrimental effects that alcohol has on our health and society as a whole, and it's done little to change people's habits. So when compelling narratives and medical benefits of cannabis surface, why do those with a different view continue to act like stubborn toddlers and ignore them?

Speaking of toddlers, marijuana has been around since we first discovered growing things could be useful to our survival. Although its first use was mainly for its strong fibre (hemp products are a versatile and useful material to this day), it wasn't long before people started ingesting it either accidentally (through the smoke of burning crops), or on purpose (through careful extraction). Cannabis has been used in various ways for thousands of years, and its seeds were traded all over the world. It's been used for various medicinal purposes, and continues to be used as a sleep aid, a treatment for glaucoma, for decreasing nausea, stimulating the appetite in cancer patients, easing anxiety, and as an analgesic for those living with chronic pain. Because of its psychoactive properties and the superstitious nature of our primitive brethren, in some cultures it was given religious-like fascination and revered as a "magical" remedy for physical and mental ailments.

These days caffeine is the most commonly used, legal psychoactive substance in the world. Besides coffee and tea, caffeine is found in everything from soda to chocolate and pain relievers, yet no one considers it drug abuse to ingest large, unregulated amounts of it. Coffee is the only drug I get to brag about using.

Caffeine is considered a psychostimulant, increasing mental alertness and the ability to concentrate, reducing fatigue, and even causing a state of mild euphoria. It can even be medicinal, constricting blood vessels to the brain to help headaches, promoting bronchial relaxation to treat asthma-like symptoms, and stimulating the drive to breathe in premature babies. It causes you to pee more and often helps people poop. It remains popular for enabling long periods of intellectual concentration without causing the loss of motor activity or coordination issues that alcohol is famous for. How many times have you watched a movie or TV show where the characters are up researching through the night and one inevitably says "I'll make more coffee?"

Like all drugs, users find that at some point their usual dose no longer gets them through the day as it once did, and coffee addicts inevitably reach for that second cup. Then a third cup. Then a fourth cup. When we become dependent on something, we start to feel bad without it and become addicted to the effects it has on us, relying on it to get us through what we need to do on a daily basis.

I once sat across from a man at Starbucks who volunteered to tell me that he was falling asleep while driving and needed to stop in regularly for his double espresso to make it home. Is this the sign of an addiction? Who's to say? You could argue he's using the caffeine as a tool for a specific purpose (a noble one too if you consider he's trying not to fall asleep behind the wheel and cause an accident), but because it's so common in our culture, we conveniently don't think of it as the performance-enhancing substance that it is.

Like alcohol, caffeine's effects have been studied and there are well known withdrawal effects: headaches, fatigue, difficulty concentrating, and negative mood (the clinical term for miserable) are all common. As a stimulant, heavy consumption of caffeine can cause anxiety or nervousness, agitation, tremors, and an increased workload of the heart—which is risky for people who already have high blood pressure or abnormal heart rates. Believe it or not, there's even such a thing as caffeine poisoning, albeit very rare.

Speaking of coffee and caffeine, let's briefly mention its more sober cousin, tea. Certain teas can also contain caffeine, and in certain cultures it's revered for its medicinal properties. Notice a theme? Our friend chamomile (a plant that has been brewed into a tea for centuries) is often used as a sleep aid, for treating fevers and colds (due to its anti-inflammatory properties), for stomach upsets and as a muscle relaxant. Apparently, it can even be used to treat haemorrhoids.

Next we have nicotine. Just as THC is the active ingredient of marijuana, nicotine is the active ingredient of tobacco, which is typically smoked via cigarettes. As another stimulant that's been used and abused by society, it too follows a familiar historical pattern. Tobacco was once used to treat various ailments such as headaches and colds, and was often praised for its medicinal properties. Cigarettes were even recommended by doctors in the US until a clear link between tobacco products and lung cancer was made in the 1950s.

Tobacco increases blood flow to the area of the brain that mediates arousal and reward, stimulating positive motivation and the relaxation of muscles—a calming, anti-anxiety effect. This accounts for the reason you'll hear (and see) smokers eager to light up in an effort to de-stress. When smokers first start smoking tobacco, the nicotine activates dopamine receptors in the brain which causes a pleasurable feeling. Over time, these receptors become desensitised and, paired with the strongly addictive properties of nicotine, users often no longer smoke for the pleasure it brings, but primarily to avoid or relieve withdrawal symptoms. It's a vicious cycle, and nicotine quickly makes users its bitch. It's a cruel, ugly shrew that siphons your money and increases the workload for your heart and your blood pressure, leaving sticky deposits of plaque in your arteries as a ticking-time-bomb to a heart attack. According to the WHO, as a carcinogen (cancer-causing agent) tobacco kills up to half of its users, and millions of those exposed to second-hand smoke.

The mass societal shift away from tolerating tobacco and cigarettes due to negative health effects is promising, and views have changed (for the most part) from a time when it was considered cool to smoke. Because of the awareness smoking tobacco has on your health, I believe people have developed a general hate-on for marijuana by association, as it's commonly depicted as being smoked like a cigarette.

What about other legal drugs? Thousands are available that were designed by pharmaceutical companies and approved for public consumption. People take medications every day to deal with a plethora of illnesses, and there is every kind under the sun: anti-inflammatories, antihistamines, antipsychotics, decongestants, narcotics, anaesthetics, muscle relaxants, steroids, hormones, calcium channel blockers, contraceptives . . . even drugs to regulate your bowel movements. In the United States, deaths from prescription drug overdoses continue to rise, particularly with the use of benzodiazepines (known commonly as tranquilizers) and opioids (used to treat moderate to severe pain). As it stands, there have been no reported deaths from a direct overdose of marijuana. It's apparently quite difficult to overdose on THC, and a lethal amount is difficult to specify since it would depend on a person's weight or size. A report from the WHO in 2018 surmises that for a 70 kg (154 lb) human, 4g would be sufficiently lethal, but in all likelihood, the user will pass out before getting there.

Lethal overdose is virtually impossible due to the absence of cannabinoid receptors (the ones THC bind to in order to do their thing) in our brain stem, which is responsible for our breathing reflex. Numerous deaths have been *associated* with the drug, due to THC detected in post-mortem toxicology reports, and stipulation regarding the side effects associated with increased heart rate, lung damage, and mental health effects. It cannot be denied that its danger is directly proportional to the effect on a person's mind, inhibiting their ability to think clearly and make safe decisions. More likely, cannabis can be lethal when it sets the stage for accidental fatalities, especially when combined with other drugs, which is often the case.

The truth is, legal or illegal, any drug can be abused and no drug is completely harmless or without possible long term effects. Oxygen—part of the very air we breathe—is considered a drug in the medical community and is toxic to premature newborns at unregulated levels. As organisms that metabolize oxygen to survive, the human body produces "reactive oxygen species" (chemicals) as by-products. The theory of oxidative stress suggests that these chemicals cause damage to our cells over time, which ultimately leads to aging and death. Basically, this suggests that humans can only live as long as we do because breathing oxygen degrades our bodies over time.

When compared to alcohol or nicotine, the most used and abused drugs in history, marijuana's intoxicating effects seem quite mild.

14
Smoking Pot:
The Basics

I use the terms cannabis and marijuana interchangeably, but it's still referred to as many other things: pot, weed, ganja, reefer, grass, chronic, Mary Jane. As a plant, it's part of the *Cannabaceae* family, which includes hemp. The two most popular sub-species of cannabis, sativa and indica, both contain THC (Tetrahydrocannabinol) which is the psychoactive chemical responsible for feeling high. Generally speaking, sativa is tall with thin leaves (the image pictured in most marijuana paraphernalia), is associated with a "head high" which affects the mind and one's mood. It can increase focus, promote creativity, and stir the imagination by imbuing menial activities with a sense of wonder and awe. Indica is short with fatter leaves, and evokes a "body high" that has a more relaxing, sluggish effect, which can enhance visceral sensations and a deeper connection to one's physical body.

There are many accessible sources and pieces of literature that can explain the mechanics, history, and progression of marijuana over time better than I ever could, and in full disclosure, I don't pretend to be a scientific expert on the inner workings or biological and chemical processes occurring with the use of marijuana. My experience is entirely subjective, and it's the psychedelic effects that interest me. Part of the allure of getting high is being able to succumb to the pleasures of our own minds and bodies amidst all the noise and lights. Escapism *is* a very real part of drug use; trying to retreat to an area of the mind that is primal and automatic can be soothing to an overactive brain.

According to the Drug Enforcement Administration (DEA) and the National Institute on Drug Abuse (NIDA) in the United States, marijuana is classified as a psychoactive (mind-altering) drug which, at its best, causes "merriment" or happiness, disinhibition, relaxation, enhanced sensory perception, and heightened imagination. At its worst, it can cause impaired judgement, disoriented perception, and coordination problems, with high doses sometimes inducing hallucinations, delusions, and paranoia. Although it can depend on the situation, mood is initially elevated, accompanied by a sense of tranquillity, before an eventual evolution into drowsiness and sedation. I like to think of this as a shift between hilarity and contemplative silence.

Different strains of cannabis are often created to isolate certain desirable effects, however, as "mother-strands" (the original parent behind the various results of replication), sativa and indica are not mutually exclusive, and both mind and bodily effects can exist concurrently as part of a high. Nowadays, the plant has been genetically altered and experimented with so much to provoke certain highs that it's hard to know if any true separation between the two exists in physical form. With the amount of experimentation that has been done over time to isolate certain desirable effects of the drug, the potency of the cannabis available today is much more precise than what it was in our grandparent's generation. Thankfully, all the in-breeding seemed to turn out better than it did for the English monarchy.

It can be common not to feel a high from ingesting cannabis the first few times, which can be due to a couple reasons. For one, there is a need to learn how to perceive it, much like The Force in *Star Wars*:

Concentrate you must, young stoner. Patience you must have. Calm you must remain.

Other aspects, like the technique of smoking and how to inhale are a barrier to perception, which I can say was an obstacle for me. Having never smoked before, I may have been too caught up in the mechanics in order to notice if I was getting high. Not knowing what to expect paired with an increased vigilance makes it a problem to perceive what being high even is. How you ingest it (if you even smoke it at all) also rolls the dice on a bunch of different factors influencing how you experience it.

I found it difficult to find consistent numbers in research that confirm how much THC actually gets absorbed into your body depending on how it's ingested. As restrictions ease concerning the use and distribution of cannabis, many new products have become available. Although smoking the buds of plant may be the most familiar, it may no longer be the most popular, with the emergence of edibles, oils, and resins. Joints (ground cannabis wrapped in rolling paper and smoked like a cigarette) are the most recognizable way to partake. Generally, they're smoked differently than tobacco cigarettes, with larger puffs taken and held for longer in the lungs to enhance the effect of the drug. The psychoactive effects can occur almost immediately after smoking and usually last between one to three hours. Even when the effect of the high wears off, the drug can be detected in the body up to twelve weeks or ninety days later depending on your level of use. This is because THC loves fat. THC clings to the fat molecules in our bodies and can take an average of two to four hours for HALF of it to get flushed out. Because it takes so long to eliminate it from our bodies, physical symptoms and affected cognitive functions (particularly memory) can last for days after smoking marijuana.

Having entered the world of pot through joint-initiation, I was inclined to pursue this medium before venturing into the various alternatives. I could never seem to master the technique of rolling a joint myself, despite being shown dozens of times and an emphasis on "establishing the draw hole," as one of Adam's friends used to tell me. Even though rolling papers are easy enough to come by, I always ended up goading Adam or Jem to roll for me, having neither the patience nor the inclination to improve. When I wanted to get high, I wanted to rush into my "chill" without getting frustrated over my poor technique. Graduating from a recreational marijuana user to "stoner" in a blur, I couldn't have them rolled fast enough, especially when my appetite was increased. By then, I decided it was a good time to go and get my own tools of the trade.

15
Tools of The Trade

When I wasn't just hoping to be at the right place at the right time or pleading with others to roll joints for me, I had been sharing Jem's one-hitter. For context, a one-hitter is a small metal or glass pipe that looks similar to a cigarette, only it's hollow inside. One end has a wider opening to pack the weed in, while the other has a small hole for you to suck from. It's like smoking a reusable joint, and because it doesn't hold as much bud or burn as long, you end up cram-packing it so you can get high with just one light.

One light + One hit= One-hitter.

Jem's holder was polished wood, as big as a pack of cards, and small enough to conceal in the palm of her hand. The top swivelled out on each side revealing two long compartments: one to store the ground flower and the other spring-loaded with the pipe. These are great tools but they don't have the freshness of a joint, and unless you clean it regularly, it can taste like the ashy residue of a cigarette.

Another tool, the grinder, is essential for all your cannabis needs. For Jem and I to get the most out of "our" one-hitter, we wanted to jam pack that pipe with as much green as possible, and this was only possible when the bud was shaved into small pieces. Sure, we could have used scissors, but we weren't barbarians.

Grinders have a minimum of two movable parts screwed together to separate the different compartments. The bud usually goes on the top tier and gets crushed by the metal pegs that hug each other when it's turned, leaving the smaller bits to drop to the level below. Usually there's another layer to the grinder with a fine mesh, where bits small enough to pass through can fall. These bits concentrate into a crystal-line brown powder which, as you can imagine, have a more potent effect. I never focused too much on smoking this, but enjoyed the stories Jem told me about how she was desperate after her supply was depleted, and packed all the crystal she could in her pipe. She spent the remainder of her night attempting to count the stucco on the ceiling of her room.

It goes without saying that smoking is proven to be awful for the lungs, and although much of the focus is placed on tobacco and cigarettes, smoking anything can cause serious health issues. For this reason, vaping has become a popular alternative to smoking because it uses heat instead of an open flame to light a substance. Using a heating system to dehydrate a product allows for a vapour to be released instead of smoke, containing less harmful chemical material. Vapour is like the heat you see from a pot of boiling water: less dense, and with little to no smell.

Vaping is a loop-hole when it comes to smoking. It allows less bud to be used while still allowing the psychoactive components to be inhaled without the nasty smoke by-products. It's also more discreet and decreases irritation to the lungs which—when no longer there—can actually make it easier to take in more THC than intended. Advocates of this form report a "cleaner, more defined" high, which is an attractive prospect to the health-conscious hypocrite like myself.

Jem and I had our first experience with vaping one afternoon when we ventured to a popular vaping lounge in the city, feeling like a couple of newly minted teenagers eager to pop our collective cherries. The lounge was conveniently located above a specialty shop for marijuana paraphernalia which, during the time before legalization, obligingly placed disclaimers on their products, stressing "for legal use only" (wink wink, nudge nudge.)

Walking up the short, steep flight of stairs to the left of the store entrance, a small booth was roped off to guard the transparent entrance to the wonderland. If the intent was to be discreet, it was pathetically ineffective and acted like a small fence overlooking the animals at a petting zoo. Jem and I weren't high at this point, so we tried to take in the atmosphere as we waited for the guy behind the counter (who was oblivious to our presence) to stop talking to the person beside him so we could be granted entrance.

To our right was a 60-inch mounted TV surrounded by its smaller brethren lining the walls, and each was playing some variation of a music video. Groupings of worn, black plush couches overcrowded the space, leaving only a small aisle to travel through. These couches were sparsely filled with bodies, groups of young adults grazing in a haze of smoke hanging in the air, their faces transfixed on the movement of the screens in front of them.

Behind the small entrance desk toward the back of the building there were tables and chairs arranged in an open layout, creating the opposite effect as the front. The space resembled a café with its rounded bistro-like tables and light, delicate chairs. At the table closest to us there was an Asian boy with glasses who was reading a book on his lap, his pocket vapourizer sitting casually on the tabletop in front of him. Eventually the warden barring our path rolled his head far enough around to spot us, and his eyes glazed over like a mounted deer head.

"Ten bucks," he said, managing to finally push air between his lips. The cover charge was unexpected, but Jem and I eagerly fished through our wallets and pushed two bills toward the hanging limb at his side. The palm of his hand was open and expectant, but the hand didn't seem willing to hold itself out far enough toward us. I imagined his grunt of acquiescence as he left us to pass through the cheesy turnstiles out onto the floor beyond.

The lounge was B.Y.O.W (bring your own weed) because it was still illegal to purchase in Canada, and it was frowned upon to ask if/where you could buy it from the staff or patrons. If you had your own supply through whatever means, this was a place you could come to borrow a device to smoke, find a spot to indulge, or buy whatever chocolate bar, chips, gum, or beverage you would eventually crave. We walked past the tables and chairs of the pseudo-café toward the far-right corner of the building, where a pavilion was set up to dispense tools and food. I was impressed by the variety of snacks they had available; it was a tactical business advantage to exploit the lazy and hungry.

Jem and I decided to rent a stationary vapourizer called the "Volcano," and had it brought over by an employee to teach us the basics. There were minimal instructions: Load the bud, turn the heat up, the bag fills with vapour, and you suck through the nipple at the end of the bag. Despite the intimidation it was exciting, and luckily, the apparatus was easy for Jem to figure out.

The taste was the first thing we noticed. While the heat of the vapour in my mouth was subtle, it had an essence of popcorn, and although it was weird, it wasn't altogether unpleasant. It started a lot like my first experience because I was convinced I wasn't getting high–focusing as hard as I was on whether I could feel anything–but this time it hit sooner. It felt lighter, like a soft high with a calming effect, as opposed to the usual harshness of a wibbly-wobbly smoking high. Without the irritating smoke as feedback, it was difficult to gauge how much we had actually consumed, and out of habit, I felt I needed to keep taking more in to get a good high. Unlike smoking from a bong, there was no harsh burn or an off-balancing wave that let me know I should probably stop to take a breather.

Jem and I sat on one of the worn black couches, sucking and passing the balloon back and forth between us. We grew oblivious to the discomfort of performing an illicit activity within a group of strangers quickly, and began to enjoy the new experience. Mesmerized by the gyrating figures on the television screens like the crowd among us, I could see how easy it would have been to spend all day there smoking, munching, and sinking into those couches, but even so, we felt out of place. Jem had an ability to adapt to social situations easier than I did, but she, too, preferred the intimate setting of our bachelorette pad, so we didn't end up staying long. Once the novelty of the vapourizer wore off and we felt like we had plateaued in our level of high, we returned the equipment, peeled ourselves off the couch, and left without so much as a snack to go.

Another method of consuming cannabis is with a bong. I must admit, with no euphemism intended, that I was initially intimidated by them. However, when it was time for me to graduate from cigarette look-alikes and one-hitters to the tools of a seasoned stoner, I found myself up to the task. Like Dr. Frankenstein, my pursuit of knowledge was exaggerated and all-encompassing; whatever the consequences, I was ready to bastardize nature, and harness the power of the four elements to feed my obsession. Jem's boyfriend Mike had recently purchased a fine stallion: an emerald green glass bong about ten inches in length, which (in true gentleman fashion) he had bequeathed to her/us. It was a little advanced for us just starting out, as neither of us really knew how to handle it (*snort*), but once we loaded it up and put our mouths to work, with a little practice, the rest came naturally (*chortle*).

A bong is a large pipe—usually glass—with a shallow amount of water filled in the bottom. In the hole at the bottom, there is space for a removable mini pipe called the downstem which is used with a "bowl" that either comes attached or separate, and the bowl is where you put the cannabis. To use it, you cover the opening of the bong with your lips resting inside, and use a lighter on the bud until it starts to burn. While it takes a bit of practice, the idea is to inhale at the same time the weed burns, so that the smoke gets pulled into the water chamber where it makes a neat bubbling noise and cools down. Once there is enough smoke trapped, you remove the downstem/bowl combo to suck in fresh air, allowing the smoke to travel up through the pipe and into your mouth. The longer you can hold your breath with the smoke in your lungs, the harder you get hit with the effects of a high.

Like a mad scientist, taking a bong hit moves you forward from theory to practice, as you harness the powers of earth, fire, water, and air in succession. One minute your head is cast down in a focused position, carefully balancing your instruments to maintain the dexterity required for the perfect execution, and the next you are pulling your mouth away from a cloud of smoke shouting "Eureka!" as new revelations hit you with the speed and force of a dump truck. It's a head-rush, and a strong and heady experience that brings you mouth-to-brain with THC's psychoactive properties. You get a faster, more intense high, and I've found the rush allows my creative juices to flow more freely despite an umbilical tether to the couch. I do, however, associate bong hits with a 50-50 outcome because of the fine line between euphoria and sheer terror. Regret can be instantaneous when it goes bad, and after you create it, it's hard to undo. Being really, really high will give you an awareness of your body that you may not wish you had.

16

The Downside

It should go without saying that mind-altering substances should be taken seriously. The mind can very quickly become a battlefield under psychedelic control, traitorously leading you from empowerment into a full-blown panic attack. I've become terribly, uncomfortably aware in a severe high. My teeth have been itchy. My gums and lips have felt so foreign that they were like two worms sliding together, and my mouth has felt like it was stuffed with cotton from being so dry and rough.

Functions that are usually filtered by your unconscious, primitive brain can become a focal point when you're psycho-activated, and an awareness of your own mortality can become unavoidable when you can't help but focus on the autonomic processes we don't usually think about, like your heartbeat and breathing. Combine that with a healthy dose of paranoia and you start to feel like you could be dying. It is possible to control this—it's the epitome of mind over matter—but the experience is not for the faint of heart.

In my early days of smoking, I was fearless and eager for these experiences, but sometimes they were positively frightening. When my fingers managed to find their way to my neck, they lingered there, feeling the artery pulse steadily, and I became hypnotized by the rhythm:

Lub Dub. Lub Dub.

The valves opened and closed, and my life's blood pushed through the ventricles of my heart. If I focused on it, I could feel each individual beat as if I could see it happening, and then, things began to slow down. I suddenly became aware of my breathing, and realized I had been holding my breath as I remained still to focus on my heartbeat.

My heart seemed to race and relax simultaneously as adrenaline surged in response to my panic, and I desperately tried to regain control of my breathing to oxygenate my body. The terror made me feel faint, and while the prospect of succumbing seemed innocent, it was overlapped with a fear that I may die if I didn't fight against it. My anxiety was a survival instinct that revived me, and the loss of control might have been more terrifying if I wasn't already familiar with it; like any of my anxiety attacks, I knew I just had to ride it out and reassure myself I was safe.

Control was, and still is, a major factor in my experience with cannabis, as I would caution it to be for anyone poking around at the old upstairs motherboard: one crossed wire and the whole thing shuts down. Depending on how hard your hit is, good *and* bad is intensified. It can make you tired and useless or happy and joyous depending on the strain and your state of mind at the time. When used with other substances—particularly the trifecta of alcohol, nicotine, and caffeine—the combination of intoxicants can be especially terrifying.

Under the lull of a high, it feels natural to want to engage in familiar vices like a cigarette or a nice cup of coffee, and living wholly in the present under the influence of cannabis, it's easy to forget how other substances can compound and overlap in your body. While I have distractedly puffed on one of Jem's cigarettes out of curiosity, I've never smoked a whole cigarette, so I can't offer subjective insight as to how it interacts with a high. Both caffeine and marijuana increase your heart rate, and I can attest that drinking coffee and smoking weed together makes me uncomfortably aware of my heart and its beating within my chest (see above).

One Halloween I had the worst experience of my life mixing marijuana with alcohol. A handful of friends and I went to a house party of a recent acquaintance, and despite an intention to make a good impression, I drank too much of those notoriously sugary alcohols that always leave you in a bad way. At some point, I overheard a few of the guys saying they were going outside to smoke a bong, and not being one to pass up an opportunity to get high, I followed them out to the front porch.

The holder of the weed was a young guy, tall and burly in a big teddy bear sort of way, and part Native American as he later told me, so it stands to assume that he had some good shit. Being the only girl in the circle of the three, I think they were a little surprised that I took to the bong like a natural and puffed away. The stuff was intense, and I probably would have enjoyed it more if I hadn't already been tipsy on alcohol. Although things went well enough as we chatted in our circle, having innocent heart-to-hearts about our lives and dreams, once we went back inside, things got sour real quick.

One of the hosts had a pet chameleon and had brought it out to show everyone. I was well gone, staring at its shifty eyeballs and forked feet, but still enough of myself to think it was adorable. I should have known it was a bad idea when one of my friends (who, whether sober or not, would have engaged in such an activity) decided to eat some live chameleon food (aka mealworms). I caught his eye, and he looked at me as if to say, "I dare you."

I dared—and I did. The worms were small enough that I reasoned I could put them out of their misery quickly, and they didn't taste like much of anything to be honest; all crunch and no bite.

In the artificial light of the basement apartment, things soon intensified as the faces of my friends pulsed in and out in a ripple between my reality and a nightmare. I became extremely aware of every internal and external nuance in the present and grew more paranoid by the moment. The panic set in, along with a terrifying realization deep in my soul that I was not prepared for this.

I tried to fight the onset of tunnel-vision and the pinpoint focus that you experience right before you faint. I knew that if I didn't fight it, I would lose consciousness, and I feared not waking up. I knew my body was trying to shut down from all of the mental and physical over-stimulation to reset. It was a safety mechanism created by the mind; when the rush of adrenaline wears off and mental exhaustion kicks in, an error message appears stating:

You have exceeded your GB limit, proceeding further will result in damage to the storage device.

I had been sitting on the couch within my new social circle, looking back and forth at the faces surrounding me. Some were familiar and others weren't, but each had a personality that soon became grotesque and cartoonish the longer I stared, so I fought tooth and nail to keep my mind moving. I was so uncomfortable that I felt like I was giving birth, and each movement was a contraction that sent me spiralling danger-ously toward shut down. Not wanting to embarrass myself in a room full of strangers or worry the friends I knew, I pulled myself together enough to take refuge in the bathroom. I closed the door behind me and opened the connection between mouth and stomach. The mental and physical overload proved to be too much, but I hadn't known what I was doing to myself until it was too late. I retched until there was nothing left, and I hugged that sweet, forgiving porcelain God, feeling his cool kiss on my cheek.

There will be varying degrees of three reactions to this story: Some may empathize, having gone through a similar experience, others will feel pity. The remaining ones will scoff, thinking something like "serves her right" or "she got what she deserves dabbling in drugs," wholly missing the point. I can assure you this slap on the wrist didn't go unheeded, but you would be remiss if you thought my story is unique. I've always liked that saying about only throwing stones at people if you can prove you're unblemished. Take a look in the mirror and tell me you've never done something you weren't proud of. The trouble is, regardless of precautions, we all still make stupid decisions as adults, teenagers, and everything in between. That's just a part of life.

This sheds light on a troubling trend in society when it comes to the benevolence we bestow on our most vulnerable. Children seem to be at the top of the list, and it's natural to try and protect them from the bad in the world. Even so, there's an invisible line that all children cross, and once they cross this line, they are lumped in with everyone else to be labelled and judged. As adults, they can become all the cruel names we use to scare the fresh meat: lowlifes, losers, scum, addicts, useless, poorly-developed. Collectively, we separate and shun others with such blatant hypocrisy as if none of us have skeletons in our closets. Without noticing, the outcasts become our most vulnerable, but when they aren't cute anymore, we don't seem to care.

When we feel alone or unhappy, we try to dull the pain. This is what leads to indulgences. Admit it, sometimes it feels good to trigger the happy hormones when we're overwhelmed with an extra piece of cake, a puff of a cigarette, a casual wank, a nice glass of wine, or even an online purchase. I'm of the opinion that if we didn't allow ourselves this every once and a while, we would go mad. If, however, the trigger to the need for these indulgences isn't addressed, addiction can form. We are *all* addicts to something, we just don't realize it, and because the word has such a negative connotation, we won't admit it even when we do. There is even the very real addiction of pretending you aren't addicted, because society picks and chooses which addictions are acceptable, changing them over time.

When it comes to the common sins like smoking and drinking too much or partying too hard, it's true that sometimes we don't know what we're doing to ourselves before it's too late. Even something as simple as the choice to avoid sunscreen and bake in the sun can have long term consequences you aren't aware of at the time. By indulging, you don't always grasp the concept of living into the consequences of our actions. We blurt whatever comes out of our mouths with no filter. We have unprotected sex because it feels better. We stay up all night watching videos on YouTube and forget we have to work the next day. The reason the elderly are wise is that they've survived their stupid shit and lived to warn others.

Although I hate myself for saying it, sometimes I think it's ok to embrace the YOLO life. Everything can kill you these days: You eat too much, you die. You drink too much, you die. You take too many of those pills meant to stop you from killing yourself—you can die that way too. We live a double-edged life, with finite bodies and infinite minds. These minds have been able to create from both sides of the spectrum; deadly toxic weapons that can obliterate millions of lives or cunning medical advances that can save them.

We live in an age where we can keep people alive longer than ever before with things like harvested organs and mechanical implants. With biotechnology we have the ability to let machines breathe for us and keep our hearts beating as they lay on a table next to us, separated from our body. Even with my experience in health care, when I watched the medical drama *Grey's Anatomy* while high, I found myself looking at the patients in the intensive care units in the episodes—with their limp bodies and spaghetti tubing linking their lives to machines—and found myself wondering if it was an abomination or a miracle that was taking place.

Life and death define our existence. What is the meaning of life, and why do we exist? What happens after we die? Our mortality is both feared and revered, but despite how we try to survive otherwise, human beings cannot escape the fact that we all have expiration dates. We live desperately trying to find meaning before our time is up, but is it possible we could be taking life a bit too seriously? Sadness and happiness may seem to be at opposite ends of a spectrum, but experiencing both rounds out the experience of existence. If we live trying to escape our feelings and our fears, are we missing the bigger picture of what it means to be alive?

17
Insights On Addiction And Restriction

It's important to have a sense of humour. Scientists have proven that laughter releases endorphins, or "feel good" brain chemicals that can decrease stress, which is often why you hear people say laughter is the best medicine. (Robin Williams personified this method of care as *Patch Adams* in a role he was born to play.) It's an interesting phenomenon to see how mental illnesses like depression are prevalent in comedians—there's something about experiencing the depths of suffering and wishing for no one to experience it as you do. For those who learn to laugh through the pain, I think there's an intelligence that reflects a kind of altered perception which is crucial to spiritual growth.

One of the great comedic geniuses and social critic, the late George Carlin, was known for his relentless and sardonic style. He was clearly intelligent and introspective, having written several published works on his craft and musings. Carlin was also an avid drug user in his younger days, as he reflects in many interviews. Self-identifying as a rebel with an anti-establishment mentality, he began smoking marijuana at age thirteen, and was a professed "stonehead" for thirty years. In an interview with *Playboy* in 1982, Carlin admitted that his daily toking routine had been slowly decreasing of its own accord, and that as much as pot had helped him through a strict Irish-Catholic etiology, he felt there was an inverse relationship between pleasure and pain that came from its constant use. He called pot a value-changing drug that "opens doors of perception," allowing you to see things differently, and expand naturally. His is a wonderful example of how cannabis can be used as a tool for personal growth; with sufficient intellect, as Carlin put it, you can realize the growing imbalance between pleasure and pain, and adjust your actions accordingly by giving up the things that hurt you.

My vision for cannabis users is different from the classic image of Bob Marley taking a hit and laughing, carefree of consequences and repercussions. Honestly, the image of a pothead is far from a flattering one. Although weed culture seems to favour liberation, peace, and freedom to be yourself, the images we're presented with are dumb, hungry, slow-moving primates who lounge around in a useless haze of smoke. I often get angry by the common stereotype of stoners in society.

A TV segment I watched about medical marijuana users focused on a shot of a person taking a hit from a vapourizer, obscuring their face in a white haze of smoke so big that it was comical (while most vapourizers produce little to no smoke, it depends on the level of heat used). No wonder people get offended by the idea that this may become common-place with legalisation, since the dangers of second-hand smoke are so well known now. Many gather in a delinquent mass on April twentieth (420) which is a date of historical significance for pot smokers, of which its origins remain hazy; there are many theories, but the most reliable indicates it was a meeting time used by a group of teens who, calling themselves "the Waldos," met to smoke pot and search for a fabled cannabis plant in California. When people try to "stick it to the man" by lighting up and sucking back theatrically-large doobies, how can we expect to be taken seriously? It explains why medicinal users don't want to be lumped in with the recreational ones.

I get it. Honestly, the world wouldn't function if everyone was high. The economy would suffer because no one would understand or accept the concept of money, thinking we could prosper on good vibes alone.

In a perpetually high society, we would decimate the world's food supply in a matter of years and damage the Earth beyond repair with our callous regard for waste (or simply the lack of energy to dispose of it properly— what is "properly" after all?). Considering all we have already done to the environment, I already believe Ms. Terra Firma is trying to kick us off her back like a gluttonous tick, swelled to the point of annoyance.

Our health care system would fall apart even further than it already has, because if our minds were only focused on the present, we would live hard and die young, losing all insight on prevention. We would sit around, glued to surfaces, pondering the meaning of life, exploring the depths of our minds and accomplish very little in the physical world. Even though they already exist, there would be a very real danger from those in society who believe they can function quite efficiently when high.

I know those who, much to my dismay, have driven while high, arguing that they are able to see hazards before the brain can even process them, which allows them to react quicker. Since the beginning of the twentieth century, many studies have been done on this topic to prove that this isn't true. Marijuana does mess with your perception after all, and the risk of being in an accident (car or otherwise) is shown to significantly increase after cannabis use. It takes longer to process things, and even reading signs can be an embarrassingly challenging task.

I was only walking when I once misinterpreted a "Please Drive Slowly" sign; the picture of a cartoon turtle smiling on it sent me into immediate panic, believing this meant there was a turtle crossing. Looking frantically at the bottom of my shoes, I dreaded the sickening crunch that would indicate my involvement in the demise of a baby turtle. Could you imagine if I were driving? The simple misperception could have prompted me to slam on my brakes suddenly, and the way other drivers in Toronto sniff your bumper so hard convinces me we all would have walked away with more than just a peck on the behind.

I know people who go to work high, arguing that their monotonous tasks in the trades are made more tolerable. Can you imagine going to work high? How could one focus and try to be productive with their mind being distracted by the intricacies of how to load a stapler? In my opinion, these choices are foolish and dangerous, but I do also believe that cannabis affects people differently.

The acute effects that cannabis has on our brains have been studied to an extent, and no doubt the substance affects our brains in more ways than we know. Unfortunately, it's difficult to get clear scientific answers, and the ones we do get are often cock-blocked by cultural stigma or biased politicians. That being said, we are coming to an age where more studies are being done to counterbalance all of the negativity toward marijuana and show more positive results. Even so, one negative area seems to hold true: the frequent use of the drug by young adults can cause potentially irreversible damage to the developing brain.

I'm not being a hypocrite when I say I completely understand the need to discourage youth from engaging in marijuana at a time when their minds are still developing. I was twenty-six when I started with the drug, and given my powerful experience, I think it's absolutely crucial that you have strong mental control when using a psychedelic substance.

It's an incredibly challenging task trying to figure out when the line between adult and adolescent splits, but the negative impacts of drugs on young adults are generally well known. Young adults are a group that is particularly susceptible to being influenced and making bad decisions. Research shows that the human brain doesn't finish developing until the mid-twenties with the frontal lobe (responsible for the ability to plan and make complex judgements) being the last to do so. It then stands to reason that since a significant period in brain growth is occurring during this time of exploration, discovery, and experimentation, anything taken during this time could cause detrimental effects to our development. Although it's usually the drugs and illegal substances that get the spotlight, many scientific studies explore the effects of unavoidable factors, such as negative childhood experiences, stress, and even sleep deprivation on brain development.

Scientific evidence suggests that prolonged use of cannabis in adolescents increases the risk of psychological difficulties they may face later in life due to the tendency for THC to impair learning and memory. I experienced a bit of this, discovering that I had greater difficulty focusing on tasks when I was sober; it's like reading a whole page in a book, knowing your eyes moved over each and every word, but being unable to explain what you just read so you have to do it all over again. Even though my thoughts moved quickly when I was under the influence, they didn't always stick, and this habit bled into my sobriety. Even without the drug in my system, it felt like my mental wires had been crossed, and I had to really focus to process my thoughts. It was a learning disability, and it made me give credit to the degenerative effects of THC.

Caution is indeed warranted when it comes to adolescents and marijuana, but my least favourite argument is the one you always hear: that it's addictive or "a gateway drug". As the body develops a tolerance to the drug from consistent use, it's assumed that the user will take greater doses to gain the same pleasurable effects, which will lead to the use and abuse of more serious drugs like heroin or cocaine. Eventually the body *will* develop a tolerance (we are incredibly adaptable as a species), but this argument assumes that users will become dependent or addicted to the drug, and that a spiral into more toxic indulgences is inevitable.

Addiction has a negative connotation, not unlike the inherited stigma of labelling mental illness. Can you become addicted to weed? Of course you can, but you can become addicted to anything— including coffee and sugar. It's the feeling you associate with the use of a substance that keeps you going back for more again and again despite the consequences. If you become addicted to cannabis, you can't blame it on the plant. To play devil's advocate, what about substances that are used for medicinal reasons? If a drug is being used to achieve a state of average functioning, then it's no different from an epileptic taking their anti-seizure medication, a schizophrenic taking their antipsychotic medication, or a diabetic taking their insulin.

I didn't become addicted to cannabis, but I did come to crave a hit in the way you would reach for a cold beer at the end of a hard day of work to relax and unwind. As a previous drug-virgin, I never felt I couldn't function without marijuana, and I always planned how it would affect me in the future while determining how I could use it to its maximum benefit. For example, if I chose to smoke on a weeknight, I would cut myself off after a certain time (planning that my high would last three to four hours) so I could minimize the chance of it affecting my sleep or ability to get up the next morning for work.

Escapism is a great determinant of predicting addiction, but it doesn't always lead to addiction. It's a response to evade an unpleasant reality, but also a mechanism of emotional survival that keeps us from feeling what our brain considers a threat. My approach to weed wasn't usually about escapism, it just so happened that it was easier to release the stresses of the day when I smoked which, as a chronic over thinker, was something I struggled with. My perspective on life became clearer, and I truly felt happier and more like the self I wanted to be when I was high.

Other arguments propose that a dependence on the high that cannabis produces can result in stunted emotional and social maturity. According to philosopher Peter Geach, marijuana leads to a "pathology of the soul" and feelings of euphoria which, not honestly earned, are harmful to the developing minds of youth. We worry that teens don't take it seriously and that they don't know the damage it will cause to them later in life. We think by keeping it illegal we scare them through fear of being caught and arrested, or getting charged with an offence that will either throw them in jail or follow them the rest of their lives. Using misguided paternalism through fear-mongering is a poor substitute for education, and a poor parenting approach can often have the opposite effect than intended. Adolescents are defined by their rebellious exploits. It's like that old saying: if I tell you to think about anything *except* a purple elephant, what do you suddenly find yourself thinking about?

18

A Tool

Modern medicine continues to try and understand the mysteries of life and death, and how our bodies carry us between the two. When society is ready, stigma seems to ease as alternative therapies make what was once old new again. Merging the natural herbal practices of Eastern medicine with the science of Western medicine creates a holistic approach to health where the mind and body are a unified focus.

In the time of old wives' tales, any miraculous cure was met with speculation and when something was not understood (and/or didn't fit into what people believed), it was feared. It wasn't that long ago in humanity's history when women were accused of witchcraft from circumstance, paranoia, proclaimed "unnatural events," or a disreputable knowledge or skill. I like to believe that society has matured, using science to discover value in the strange and unusual, rather than defaulting to the herd mentality of religion to guide our rules.

A lot can be said of unconventional medicine, and the only reason it's labelled as unconventional is because it doesn't conform to the majority. Cannabis is an unconventional medicine, but it's certainly not the only plant in our medicinal repertoire that's been used to treat ailments. Aromatherapy uses the essence of flowers. The smell of lavender, for example, has been proven to promote relaxation and relieve stress. I've already mentioned our friend chamomile, but there are hundreds if not thousands of the products from the natural world that we can get over-the-counter for various ailments: St. John's-wort, witch hazel, tea tree oil, ginseng, flaxseed, milk thistle, echinacea, and gingko biloba, to name a few available at the drug store.

My ailment was psychological: depression, a lack of meaning, cynicism, pride—and the natural world provided a soothing medicine for me. Once I started smoking marijuana, the effects on my psyche were earth-shattering, and although I can't say I've ever had the kind of vision I sought when I considered trying psychedelic mushrooms, I fell into moments of powerful introspection. You could say the drug led me to a revelation: to see things that are no longer shaded by the clouds of our past experiences and that allow personal and spiritual growth.

It was a new sense of wonder at the world and the people and things within it that made me feel like I was experiencing everything for the first time. With a renewed appreciation for the mundane, I was happily baffled by things such as the engineering behind the creation of a change sorter. It was the shift in perspective that pushed getting high past a simple indulgence in escapism toward a lighter, more joyous part of life, and the realization that it's so easy to miss this joy if we don't know how (or where) to look. I felt like I had found Waldo for the first time, and I wanted to show everyone where he was.

For those who have never tried weed, I'm sure this is a difficult concept to grasp—it's all New Age and hippy-dippy—and frankly quite easy to make fun of. Simple, mind-numbing revelations are a joy of life, and a stoner staple. (*Bruh . . . If a tomato is a fruit, does that make ketchup a smoothie?*) It's true that the drug appears to dull our minds on the outside—stereotypes often have a basis in truth, after all. Although you feel inflated by a newfound ego with more distinct thoughts, verbalizing these thoughts is much slower, and you are aware of how you sound to others who are sober: slow and clearly intoxicated. There is a pang of sadness and rejection at this, learning that others can't even *try* to understand unless they've had their own personal experience.

So what can we take away from this stoner mentality? In this age of money, capitalism, and greed, it's hard to define something's worth without a physical form to exploit. If a purpose cannot be measured, it can often be difficult to fathom, and without measuring its success it becomes impossible to accomplish. It's easy as an outsider to assume the worst of a pot-smoker; that they are a smelly, morally weak degenerate. A hippie. A rebel. A coward trying to run away from responsibility. I used to think this way after all, and until I was willing to challenge my old beliefs and biases, I lived in cynical ignorance. Challenging these beliefs was a part of my self-discovery, and marijuana unlocked my subconscious to lay these oppressive thoughts bare. As they say, acceptance is the first step to recovery dontcha know.

Identifying negative patterns is one thing, but choosing to overcome them is a form of mental ascension. Controversial as it may be, I believe cannabis is a tool for this, and with the peace and wisdom that inevitably follows, we may even be able to access the soul.

The soul is immortal and transcends death, which we fear so much. Perhaps there is some merit in feelings like déjà vu or other disjointed familiarities in our present lives, which could be residual from a past one. To be able to intellectually explore the boundaries of science and spirituality is something we need to do more often, if we want to consider these answers.

Science can teach us how drugs affect our brains but cannot predict how they will affect our minds. Ever heard someone described as a happy drunk? How about an angry drunk? Although the drug of choice may be the same, our psyches are affected differently, which may shed some light on why people are drawn to use drugs, illegal or otherwise. Are some people born to be drug users? Do addictive personalities create drug users? What creates an addictive personality? These questions spark the nature versus nurture debate that psychology has been arguing for decades. Namely, how does individual experience affect us as human beings, and how do we become who we are? Do we act the way we do as a result of our genetic dispositions or from the way our environment shapes us? If we don't like what we see in ourselves, can we ever change?

Like Freud's psychological metaphor about the iceberg and subconscious, we already know that our subconscious plays a hidden part in our lives only visible beneath the surface. If we were able to bring this submerged ice up from the depths of our consciousness, perhaps we could learn to understand ourselves better. The science of psychology has always fascinated me; although the mind is abstract and infinite, the brain is physical and finite, and the connection between the two is something we have not fully been able to understand to this day.

Drawing on beliefs of mindfulness through science or spirituality, practicing meditation techniques focuses the mind on present circumstances in an effort to control our responses to them. Given the psychedelic properties of the THC in cannabis, it's this confrontation with our minds that makes me believe in its untapped potential. Of course, this kind of journey forces us to face our thoughts and because of this, it makes perfect sense why people can have "bad trips." We can get easily get carried away by our anxieties.

But what if we could harness this introspective power in a controlled environment? Just like our emotions are shaped from memories, which then shape our actions in life, what if we could create an environment that allowed us to harness the high, to come face-to-face with our fears and ultimately override them? Think about it as an adjunct to cognitive behavioural therapy, which challenges negative patterns of thought in order to alter unwanted behaviour patterns. If we can learn to control our body's response through repetitive exposure to something that makes us uneasy, with the addition of some psychoactive sugar, we have the makings of an unconventional, yet ground-breaking approach to cure phobias.

To get really philosophical, we could question the balance of neural networks that are created or destroyed from weed. Could we argue that only weaker neurons are destroyed to be replaced by stronger, augmented ones? Are these connections created in addition to, or at the expense of others? I can tell you that surprisingly, the more often I became high, the faster my brain seemed to work making connections and recognizing patterns. Despite the induced attention deficit disorder (ADD), I was able to recall past emotions and experiences rather than getting lost in their newness, which allowed me to bypass the sense of wonder and skip straight to the philosophical intelligence of what I was experiencing. In other words, new experiences felt familiar, and my reactions became informed. This is the role of our limbic system: the collection of structures in our brain involved in learning, processing emotions, and memory.

I may be delving into more science fiction than reality, like the world of the movie *Limitless,* in which a delicious Bradley Cooper finds himself under the influence of the mysterious drug NZT-48, allowing him to unlock his brain's full potential. The ruminations of a high mind go hand-in-hand with the limitless power of imagination, but it's fun to think about. Do the psychoactive properties of THC slow the mind to a point of retardation, or are we enhanced with an intellectual insight?

It may be ignorant to think we can access a higher ascension to the spiritual realm without some sort of sacrifice. I'm not talking about a face-melting sacrifice, like in *Indiana Jones: Raiders of the Lost Ark,* but perhaps just a piece of our mortal bodies; since we are mortal, we cannot survive with so much divine knowledge. Perhaps this sacrifice is like the cholesterol and plaque that slowly builds up in our arteries as we consume unhealthy foods. Perhaps the memory loss, ADD, and inability to concentrate that can come from long-term cannabis consumption are just as insidious as heart disease. Just as the heart can only compensate for blocked arteries for so long, the mind can only operate on so high a frequency for a limited time.

There is no doubt that smoking is damaging to the lungs, but I found it was the way to get the best onset and duration of the effects of THC from marijuana. Unlike edibles that can take up to an hour to kick in and peak after two to three hours, smoking allowed me to decide if I wanted to continue my high by smoking more, or sobering up. Although vaping is healthier because of the decreased amount of ash and resin being pulled into the lungs, I found I ended up vaping more frequently to reach my desired level of high. Despite the potential damage, the priceless episodes of healing that came from my indulgence makes me wonder if it all evens out in the end.

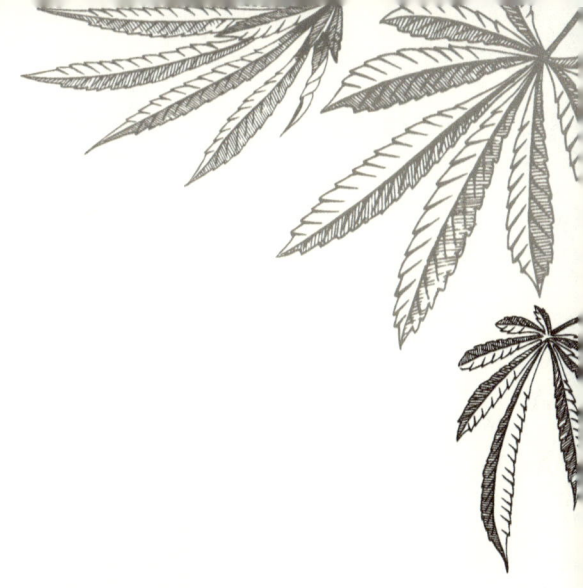

PART IV:
BODY AND MIND

19
Music

When I first decided I wanted to write about my experiences with cannabis, I tried to pin down the process of becoming high. As I used cannabis more and more, however, I realized this process could never be perfect (or even reliably accurate) due to various factors like my mood, the strain I was smoking, and my increased tolerance to the drug.

Overall, part of the fun is that experiences are fluid, constantly changing and diverging yet often coming together to meld into an abstract whole. Since we perceive reality through our senses, under the influence of a high, each is magnified in ways that make life like an amusement park: After paying your admission fare, once you step through the gate all rides are free and the lines are short.

One of the first things Adam told me to do when I got high was to listen to music. It's been suggested that music is the language of the soul, and despite the different dialects, it's universally enjoyed. I've never felt a strong connection to music in my life (something others consider a serious sin), but I've been surrounded by those who have their very identities entwined with it, brandishing their bodies in its symbols and merchandise, and travelling the country seeking concerts. I felt unable to connect with this medium of emotion that seemed to resonate with so many others, and I felt like an outcast because of it;

whereas music seemed to connect people, I was merely grateful for the background noise it provided to avoid silent car rides with my parents.

I do *like* music—there were few times in my youth when I obsessed over bands, or caught a song-bug that would last for weeks, but I never saw it as a way to express an identity the way some people (particularly the adolescent folk) do. It was really common for the men I dated to surround their lives with music. I even followed one man from concert to concert for months like a lovesick puppy, hoping to develop a similar connection to music that would ultimately allow me to become closer to him. Alas, it was to no avail.

In high school, my usual disdain for concerts and large crowds of people was overshadowed by my obsession with the band Fall Out Boy and their lead singer. When one of their tours made it to Canada, I decided I was going to go to a concert in London, Ontario, which was an hour out of town. For better or worse, fear of the unknown is muted when I'm singularly focused on a passion project. I didn't know how the conversation was going to go with my mom, but I convinced myself I was going to make it happen no matter what.

"There's a concert I want to go to," I told her one day.

"Where?" she asked, after a small pause.

". . . London. Not England."

". . . How are you going to get there?"

"GO train. I already figured out the route, but I think the trains stop before the show ends, so I was thinking of renting a hotel room for the night and coming home the next day."

I could tell she wasn't happy about that.

"I'll pick you up. Call me when it's done."

Although she didn't give me a choice, I was secretly relieved. So, after finishing a night of work at her second job as a waitress, my mom drove an hour out of town to pick me up from my first real concert.

I found my way through the city to the hub of GO trains and buses which were entangled, overlapping like spider webs, while strangers from everywhere came and went. The train ride was uneventful, and it was relatively simple to find the venue. I arrived well before the show was meant to start, but there were already people camped out, waiting in line along the concrete exterior of the building. I got in line behind three young girls about my age, and out of proximity, found myself involved in their conversation surrounding the band. It was an odd feeling for me, being so easily embraced into a group that knew little about me, but the only thing that mattered was my similar interest. We introduced ourselves, talked briefly about our experiences getting tickets, shared food, and saved each other's spot in line when one of us had to go to the bathroom.

As the sun set, both the line behind us and our excitement grew. Before we knew what was happening we were moving forward, smiling and giddy to know that the moment we had all been waiting for had arrived. We all had tickets for standing room, and in the great swell of the crowd I eventually lost sight of my new friends. They had been replaced by the mass of people around me, each of us shoulder to shoulder, pushing and prodding each other carelessly as we swayed to the music and lost ourselves in the spectacle of the show. I felt comforted by the feel of the bodies surrounding me, oddly soothed by the feel of strange skin, and seduced by the intimacy of strangers. I was surprised to find myself at ease despite the chaos surrounding me, choosing to fully embrace the feeling of being a part of a collective something, which was so at odds with my daily reality.

When I felt my Motorola flip phone vibrate in my pocket, I knew my mom had arrived to pick me up, and my time was up even though I wished I could have stayed until the very end, when the crowd had cleared. I would have stood alone facing the empty stage, surrounded by discarded confetti that littered the ground. I would have closed my eyes and imagined being in that swell of strangers again, comforted by the animosity and collective veneration for the sound that pulsed between and through us all. I would have imagined it all again, to assure myself that it actually happened.

Instead, I threaded my way through the crowd that had just started to disperse, glancing longingly at the merchandise that had conveniently materialized at the exits, to find my mom's car. I could tell she was tired when I got in, and I sensed her frustration navigating the parking lot to the exit as concert-goers swarmed around us like zombies. As we sat in our familiar silence on the trip home, I was relieved that I was going home to the comfort of my own bed. Although I felt guilty for her having to drive so far after her long day, I was secretly grateful. Even if it was out of fear for my safety, she had never tried to stop me from pursuing something that she could see was obviously important to me, and even went out of her way despite the inconvenience. I didn't intend to ever burden to her with my choices, but she remained involved in my life no matter how distant I acted. I don't know if I ever told her how much I appreciated what she did for me that night.

I never found my new friends from the concert again, but their kindness never left me, and neither did the way it felt to be so easily embraced and included. Even though it was a pivotal experience in my life, I never went to another concert. After my obsession faded, I reverted back to appreciating music without forming a connection to it.

The opposite became true when I was high. Music burst through my indifference and transformed my existence. I lived in each moment of every note, and through the sound I felt a familiar euphoria that I hadn't felt since being shoulder-to-shoulder with strangers in a concert long gone. I became one with it in a way that was unfamiliar to my sober state, and I detached from my body to float upwards as the vibrations played against my skull. The wires of my senses crossed to the point where I *felt* the sound rather than hearing it, and whatever I listened to completely absorbed and shaped me.

With the seduction of the Phantom of the Opera's "Music of the Night," I was spellbound and possessed, pulled into the phantom's dark existence underground. I was energized and transformed into a back-up dancer listening to Kiesza's "Hideaway" and soothed into nirvana by Phil Collins' velvety voice and his drum solos in "In the Air Tonight." As the female version of Johnny Cash, Lana Del Ray sang her haunted striptease through "Gods and Monsters", and the soundtrack of *Braveheart* personified an orgasm. My favourite music to listen to was mostly instrumental because of the images my mind conjured from the notes and the emotions that were invoked, but my go-to playlists on Songza (a far superior predecessor of Google Play) were oddly specific genres of randomized music like "DJ remixes of Popular Songs," "Seductive, Sweaty Ballads," or "Poppy, Catchy Songs."

Music connects the divide between thinking and feeling. The soul answers in response to rhythm in the way that we are all matter and particles, vibrating in unison to our existence. Any wall between the left and right brain seems to disappear under the influence of a high— which is perhaps why music became so poignant to my experience, as I tend to be an overthinker. There is nothing comparable to the pull of a beat drop under the influence, when any mental walls have fallen to allow the primitive lure of the music that tempts your soul from your body. For as long as I remained transfixed, I felt free to exist and move in whatever direction I was taken, shielded from any fear of judgement as I danced.

Listening with headphones amplifies the experience, but at one point I was convinced I was experiencing some sort of mental breakdown . . . hearing disjointed sound bites and haunting static for several minutes, it took longer than I care to admit for me to realize that my headphones weren't connected properly to my music device.

Basically, if you love music, the experience of listening in a high will blow you away. If you think music is just okay, like I did, the experience is like learning a new language, and it can literally change you.

20
Body

The easiest way I can think of to describe the experience of a deep, all-encompassing body high it is to relate it to the feeling of fainting. If you've been (un)fortunate enough as I have to become well acquainted with the sensation, you can empathize more deeply with the sudden tunnel-vision, heavy eyelids, and weightless feeling that makes you feel like a balloon floating off into the sky. Like getting sucked into a vortex, you can feel the spin of the earth when you close your eyes. I guess it is similar to being piss-drunk, minus the nausea, plus or minus some anxiety.

To touch and to feel are paramount to your existence, and I've never felt more in touch with my body than when I'm high. Both pleasant and unpleasant, my muscles twitch, groan, shake, and stretch when I go about my regular routine, in ways I usually overlook. When I once bent down to grab some dry kibble from the cat food bag and feed KitKat, my journey upwards trapped my muscles in a cycle of holding and releasing the tension to maintain my standing position. I stood there, arms outstretched and vibrating inwardly as I faced the wall, and I imagined two things: what kind of an idiot I must have looked like, and the patience of my cat as she sat there watching and waiting for me to get my shit together.

For this reason, yoga is amazing to do while high.

Ganja yoga emphasizes meditation, relaxation, and a 'one-ness' with your body that you've probably never felt before. Adam introduced me to the concept after telling me he went to yoga high a couple of times and enjoyed it. This intrigued me even more, because I never thought I would hear my brother say he voluntarily agreed to do yoga. I'd taken some classes before, even trying Bikram yoga (aka hot yoga), but found the desire to become more relaxed and limber was easily outweighed by the awkwardness of rolling around, trying to hold onto my slippery, sweaty limbs for an hour in a room full of strangers.

By the time Adam suggested ganja yoga, I was more comfortable outside the security of my bachelorette pad and pushing the boundaries of my comfort zone with the drug. Besides that, any way to make exercise more enjoyable was worth a shot.

I attended a class with Adam in a little studio at the back of a head shop downtown, and as we waited around for the room to be setup, the other patrons and I were left to browse the shop's wares. Nearby, two men were having an interesting conversation:

"Ya, every day I ask Spirit, 'What should I do today?' 'How are things, Spirit?' You're saying I could worry less?' 'Okay, Spirit, I'll try, thanks.'"

Between the three of us standing there (Adam had wandered off to the corner and began socializing with a few others), it was hard to believe anyone was a part of this conversation and sober. Despite the ever-opening mind I had toward spirituality, this seemed a little much for me at the time—I cringed inwardly, feeling like I had stumbled into the wrong class at school.

What is the 'Spirit' nonsense? Were we going to bang drums and sing 'Kumbaya My Lord'? Or would a Ouija board be more appropriate?

I was reminded that my shadow was alive and well, still judging others with her childish belief in superiority.

When our small group was finally allowed to enter the studio, we spread out and set up our spots in the small space. A communal Volcano vapourizer was set up in the middle of the room by the instructor, and her helpers came along and told everyone they could contribute with a nugget of weed (in retrospect, I was amused to realize we were making offerings to a volcano as a primitive culture might). I went up with my offering that Adam had advised me to bring ahead of time, and watched with a fond remembrance as the bag of the device blew up like a balloon, identical to the one Jem and I tried at the vape lounge. Once fully inflated, the balloon was passed around the room like a ceremonial pipe, and before I knew it, we were off stretching.

There is a reason a morning stretch feels so good: when you have the opportunity to expand your muscles and joints after they've been stuck in the same position for a while, they cry in relief, and honestly, sometimes a good cry is what we need to reset. I was communicating with my body, feeling the effect of every single movement I took as I tried to contort myself, guiding it to unwind. Any discomfort was pleasantly buffered by the effects of the THC in a similar way to an analgesic, allowing me to hold positions longer and deeper as I comfortably reached my threshold for pain. You always hear about the importance of breathing in yoga, and how to coordinate your stretches with your breaths. At the best of times I have trouble coordinating my feet in front of me, but as soon as the high took hold my body moved of its own accord, releasing tension that didn't even know I had created, and allowed my breath to inevitably follow in sequence.

As I sat and meditated, I also stretched the muscles of my mind with my breath. By focusing, I tightened my chest muscles before releasing them in a sigh, and the air exchange felt displaced, like I was floating instead of just breathing. I felt like I was being lifted away by a climax I hadn't yet reached, and an inner sense of tranquillity followed as I forgot about the needs of the flesh. Connecting to the deadly perfection of the universe was foremost in my mind, along with meeting this Spirit I had heard about. I pictured all the negative space in the world as an ethereal light instead of an assumed darkness.

As an exercise, ganja yoga was incredibly appealing by the lack of sweat, but I could feel my increased heart rate to know I was exercising.

It was pure organic biofeedback, and most of all it was *fun*. Being high, the anxiety around exercising with a group of strangers was gone, replaced by solid concentration on the movements and achieving a quality stretch. My focus wasn't on my embarrassment of ineptitude (as it usually is in group skill sessions), and my self-confidence was buoyed from an inflated ego which grew as the movements became easier. Mid-session we took a break to lay in savasana (also known as the easiest/I-can't-believe-this-is-yoga pose in which you lie simply on your back) and contemplated the ceiling. Some of us took another toke of the vapourized THC before we continued, and away we went again. To maximize the benefits, I made sure to have some "yoga water" (tea) for the antioxidants as an extra pat on the back for doing something healthy.

When discussing the effects of a body high, I would be remiss if I didn't mention sexuality as an important part of the experience. Although my main interest is in the mind, there is an unavoidable connection between the mind and the body, and how marijuana affects sex that cannot be ignored. As a heterosexual woman, I can only speak of my experience, but since I've touched upon cannabis's tendency to slow time down, intensify feelings, and uncover meaning in everyday tasks, I'm sure you can imagine what an orgasm would be like under the influence. In this way, it's very similar to yoga, and this awareness of the body is quite easily one of the most amazing feelings in the world.

In my humble experience, the female orgasm is just like a good stretch. You start to let your guard down long enough to follow your body's natural movements into positions that are the most comfortable. You keep working at it—being persistent enough to find the perfect spot. As you feel yourself limbering up, your movements become more fluid until time stops, and you feel yourself floating careless and free; it's a brief experience, but it personifies the saying "hard work brings just rewards." It feels a lot like that moment when you're at the top of a roller coaster: adrenaline mixed with anticipation, before you finally drop.

There are a lot of things wrong in our supposed-modern society as it relates to sexuality, particularly in the way there are "right" and "wrong" ways to express it. In the rest of the animal kingdom, all variants seem to fit in nicely: females are allowed to be the more aggressive of the species, males can be more fabulous, and it's not uncommon for herds to be both matriarchal and patriarchal. I lie awake at night questioning the double standard of our species in Western society, especially when it comes to sexuality. For some reason lesbian porn is acceptable for men, but God forbid they see another man in the picture?

It's just another man's penis dude. Relax—it's not going to steal your imaginary girlfriend.

Homosexuality is still met with gasps and head shakes and is enough to make a metrosexual man desperate to prove his hetero-normativity. Additionally, if I, a female, go to the gym and work hard on sculpting my body, then wear clothes that show it off and make me feel sexy, suddenly I'm a slut or tramp inviting unwanted attention because a man can't control his sexual impulses. If we want to boast that we are an intelligent species, isn't this blatant hypocrisy? Our society shouldn't be threatened by an inability to overcome our primal natures or the sexually divergent. Ironically, when it comes to our most natural impulses, society is the most belligerent.

I was once watching an interview with actress Malin Ackerman who was discussing how, being of Swedish heritage, she was brought up in an environment where it was normal for children to grow up seeing their family in the nude because of their propensity to use saunas. It was very interesting to listen to how she compared her experience of nudity and sexuality to that of American society's, in which these subjects come across as taboo or forbidden; this makes it more dangerously attractive to us. In some cultures it remains this way, but in Western society, it is thankfully becoming more acceptable to embrace our sexuality as part of the human experience.

Sex is an intensely personal and intimate experience to which little compares, whether you are high or not. Fuck yeah, an orgasm feels good, but I have often wondered if there was anything to take from it, or if it was simply one of many fleeting feelings life has. I've always preferred the intellectual foreplay that leads to life changes over my corporeal needs, and this was amplified when I was high. Besides feeling the movement of the earth beneath my feet, I wanted to pursue my innocent curiosity that reached toward the stars. I wanted to grow greater, beyond one person in a world of billions. And yet, despite my lofty ambitions, I often existed in the centre of my own universe, fixated on earthly pleasures.

21
Smell/Taste

Speaking of earthly pleasures, the cliché is true: eating often becomes central to a stoner's existence. I refer of course to the fabled "munchies." When high, you can develop a near-uncontrollable urge to consume. I felt like a vampire, attempting to suck the life force from food, drawing the flavours into my taste buds with a fervour akin to sensual desire. You know you're a victim to the munchies when you open the fridge looking for a snack and see food items solely for their tastes: Oh that's salty, that's sweet. That's hot, that's cold. You don't really care what it is, as long as it has the flavours you crave.

Provided it can be done safely, preparing food and cooking is just as much of a recreational activity as eating it. Common things became mesmerizing, and I never noticed how all citrus fruits (lemon, orange, grapefruit, lime) looked the same on the inside . . . or how disturbing it was to cut raw meat, peeling away the sticky, fatty layers of chicken as I sliced into the dead (but delicious) flesh. Although I don't normally consider myself squeamish, the activity was unsettling.

With my heightened senses, I was able to simultaneously smell and taste my ingredients, and the pleasure centres of my brain blurred together with everything else, allowing every nuance of flavour to be picked out. I finally discovered that the secret to an old family recipe was a fine balance between rosemary and salt—for the longest time this knowledge eluded me, and I could never figure out why my dad's version of Pasta e Fagioli was always better than mine.

As the pesky barrier separating the senses disappears, logic is dispatched from reason, and it's quite easy to trick the brain. I was once able to convince myself that the coconut yogurt and walnut pieces that I was eating was maple walnut ice cream; considering I had none of my favourite ice cream available to me, the ingredients at my disposal were close enough that all I had to do was believe. We are always our most creative when trying to fulfill a desire, and what that is can be some really weird shit and defy all manners of class, like the time I decided it would be a good idea to drop a bit of my chocolate ice cream cake into some coffee because—you know—chocolate iced coffee. My senses knew what they craved, but I just relied on instinct and created a version of a mocha. You can create the ultimate adult milkshake, as Jem and I did, by appreciating the alcohol equivalent of Neapolitan ice cream: Tequila rose liqueur (strawberry), rum (chocolate), and vodka (vanilla).

When it comes to being high and chowing down, anything goes, and certain social faux pas (like playing with your food) are understandably allowed. Do you remember those little corn chips that look like tiny horns? The ones you put on the ends of your fingertips as you pretended to have claws? Go on with your silly self! Remember when you were young and told yourself when you were grown-up you could eat whatever you wanted, whenever you wanted? Now is that time.

Eat guacamole with a spoon like a meal.

Melt real butter on your microwave popcorn.

Eat a Pop-Tart for supper—it's a well-balanced meal for a stoner: the cookie/cracker layer embraces the craving for crunch, the jelly middle caters to the desire for sweet and fruity, and the icing adds a smooth garnish of all flavours. Sprinkles are optional. This is the dream, kids!

I learned early on to never underestimate the pull of the munchies, so I sometimes try to redirect them. Fortunately, as a woman growing up in a society that focuses unabashedly on our bodies, this came natural to me. Unfortunately, junk food comes by its name honestly, and when inhibitions are lowered in the present moment, it's hard to remember that what you put into your body directly affects what you get out of it. My advice—if you should find yourself swaying high on a cloud of ganja craving something sweet and rich—is to grab some Nutella and a butter knife. Scoop that dirty butter using just the tip of the knife and have a small taste, because the experience is all your body really wants. Let it dissolve on your tongue and feel your taste buds activate as the dopamine rush hits, and when it's over take another taste, but always go slow.

If chocolate isn't your thing but you want something sweet, go for fruits. The excitement of having a bowl of frozen berries slowly melting in your lap teaches pacing and moderation. Or try a lozenge; you'd be amazed at the variety of flavours there are out there, and the calories are so minimal you could have a handful before they add up to that donut you really crave. Maybe you're really craving salt? Boil some edamame, coat them in salt, and suck until the cows come home. Applesauce is also a semi-healthy option for those craving tart.

When I was released from the control of sobriety, my simple cravings uncovered an equally primitive narrow-mindedness that was so deeply submerged in my unconsciousness—I refer to this as the "Chips and Candies Incident."

After a munchie-run to our local twenty-four-hour convenience store, Jem and I returned home with our spoils spread out in front of us on the living room table. While she opened the bag of her Sour Patch Kids, I went for one of the many bags of flavoured chips. After our tongues had been painted in the sugar and salt respectively, she reached over to nonchalantly open a bag of Doritos chips, popped a chip into her mouth, and subsequently blew my mind.

I was always the kind of gal that liked her mashed potatoes and corn separate; each thing has its own taste, which required it to have a separate place, with each nuance separated. Now, here I was witnessing the sacrilegious mix of Sour Patch Kids and Doritos: sugar and cheese, sweet and salty, opposite sides of the taste spectrum that, in my mind, didn't belong together. I was a creature of careful, self-imposed structure, and habitually I finished one snack before opening another.

Instead of disgust, I was surprised to find that I was intrigued, spurred on by the food-lust triggered in my brain. I was struck by the brilliance of a new personal freedom, and all the snacks now available to me would never had occurred to me otherwise if I wasn't high. Bolstered against the fear of change, such a simple discovery created the opportunity for growth. After I settled my inner critic, I followed Jem down the rabbit-hole of indulgence, clashing sugar and salt on my tongue with my ketchup chips and chocolate-covered almonds; each cluster of taste buds screamed in confusion but ultimately settled, placated by the attention they received. It was overwhelming but not entirely unpleasant, and even though I decided it was something I didn't care for, I was happy that I tried something new. I took solace in knowing that even the small steps I took toward change promised larger realizations.

The Chips and Candies incident was a small event that triggered my willingness to be open, and it also helped me appreciate how the joy that can be taken from the little things in life is seriously underrated. Although a psychedelic journey of the senses is difficult to convey through words, imagine for a moment, experiencing a shared moment with another person; while you feel like the most honest version of yourself in good company, the connection brings an experience that is nothing short of soul-satisfying.

One evening Jem and I had settled in for the night with the intention of ordering take-out and getting as high as a kite. In the middle of a giggle fit, surrounded by the warm evening air on our balcony, her phone suddenly rang to signal that the delivery person had arrived with our food. Absorbed in the stillness of time as we were, all thoughts of past and present had faded, and now we were thrust back into the present, having forgotten all about our order.

In an awkward state between sheer delight at the arrival of food, and pure terror that we would have to socially interact with a stranger, Jem pressed the button on her phone, allowing them into the building. We knew their ride up the elevator to our floor wouldn't be long, and their walk to the end of the hall where our unit was would be even shorter.

We quickly gathered our paraphernalia and hurdled through the balcony portal into reality, sliding the door closed behind us. As we waited, bubbles brewed in our bellies and a wave of giggles crested past our vocal cords. When we looked at each other, the mere sight of the tears forming in the corners of our eyes threatened our sanity, and as we revelled in the joy of our laughter, we fought to maintain composure. It was the kind of laughter that takes away your ability to speak, leaving only silent cries of delight that pulls your cheeks high into your eyes, forcing them to squint and close. Trying to stifle it was next to madness, and despite breathing in deep gulps of air, we were easily blind-sighted by another fit of giggles.

When time resumed for us, a knock at the door signalled showtime, and the curtains drew back on our performance. As it was her time to buy, Jem took charge and opened the door.

Act normal, damnit!

I tried to distract myself, allowing her to complete the transaction without influence, and for a couple minutes it worked—until I heard her start to crack. The surface tension in my belly broke, and the laughter threatened to boil over again.

Pull it together!

I brought a hand up to my mouth, attempting to stifle the sound threatening to escape, and tried to disappear into the wall behind me.

Hoooooooold!

I pleaded with myself, imagining a losing battle with a ship's sail in a hurricane.

Finally the transaction was complete, and Jem handed the debit card machine back to the delivery man, managing a smile—a risky move—before closing the door. We turned to each other, reflecting a shared pride when our eyes met, and burst out laughing once again while high-fives (no pun intended) ensued. Like an invisible shield, our intoxication protected us from shame at the amount of difficulty we faced trying to act normal.

When we chose not to interact with the food gods (those that mercifully deliver to us in our intoxicated state), or when funds were low, Jem and I followed a particular pattern of indulgence. As a practiced visionary, Jem prepared feasts for herself in anticipation of the hibernation that was inevitably to follow. I marvelled at the way she intuitively paired plates of various foods and tastes like savoury deli meats with salty pepperoncini (one of our favourites), or fresh fruits with chocolate dip. She repurposed whatever was left over, be it the take-out food from the night before or the donations she collected from work as the secretary at a holistic health clinic. She adapted like a squirrel, accepting donations graciously (albeit suspiciously), and then hoarding them away for darker times ahead. From this she became incredibly inventive, able to enjoy things in eccentric ways that put her on a different mental plane in my eyes. With food, she was simply able to cater to her stoned palate in ways I never could premeditate on. It was one of the many things I loved about her.

22
Entertainment

Once the hypnotic allure of our primal need to seek munchies was broken, Jem and I gravitated toward a more passive activity to feed our minds after we fed our bodies. We connected one of our laptops to the television screen and followed our distractible minds down a rabbit hole into the abyss of the world-wide web. We even made a game of it, calling them our "YouTube Parties."

Aint-no-party-like-a-youtube-party-cuz-a-youtube-party-don't-stop!

There were a few simple rules:

1. Someone goes first. This person chose a video for everyone to watch, which had to be ten minutes or less (this minimized the amount of watching time for painful videos).
2. The complete video needed to play, although we didn't hold each other accountable to watch it thoroughly. It would be judged, admired, hated, talked through, or even ignored—but it had to play completely through.
3. The other person picked the next video to watch based only on the suggestions that appeared after the one that just finished. Depending on our mood, we sometimes included related videos that were suggested in the side panel.

Each person had an opportunity to steer the entertainment toward whatever they wanted, and when it was their turn, they were in charge. The game could end wherever and whenever we wanted, and it was a fun way to include each other in a low maintenance activity to feed our minds. We reflected with awe on where we led ourselves through the internet rabbit hole, moving from completely unrelated topics like the mating habits of sharks, to a list of the top ten celebrity plastic surgery fails. It was a kind of game that everyone won and often spurred the strangest conversations. It was surprising at times, to find out what interested one another, although I often got frustrated when Jem chose to watch advertisements because I made it a regular habit to skip them.

My personal favourite corner of the internet I saved for myself: watching hunky celebrity interviews. While high, I became immersed into the live audience as if I was really there rather than watching from a screen. My empathy feelers were on fire analyzing body language and picking up on every social cue, trying to figure out who the man was behind the public persona. I have no shame admitting that I spent hours on my laptop watching interviews and clips of my favourite male celebrities in a THC-induced haze. I noticed a common trend in my choices: prominent jaw/cheek bones, scruffy facial hair, a killer sense of humour (usually self-depreciating), charismatic, a foreign accent . . .

Jem calls love an addiction, and she often told me to "find your cigarette". Well oh boy, did I. Honestly, having a crush on a "real" person can be quite disappointing, so I used my imagination to fill a void, and stitched together the nuances I liked from the tortured creativity of James Franco, the self-aware comedic intelligence of Bo Burnham, and the lurking sexuality of Michael Fassbender. I added a splash of Henry Cavill's burly physique, and topped it all off with traits from who I consider to be the most charming man in the world: Tom Hiddleston.

Hubba Hubba.

After devouring food to satisfy the internal munchie gods, Jem's eyelids often grew heavy and she fell asleep, softly snoring halfway through whatever it was we were watching (much to my annoyance). Eyelids are traitorous things: small and easy to ignore until they suddenly become the strongest muscle in your body when you are trying to stay awake. I always tried to resist their pulsing pull, but I can empathize when the seduction of a high whispers to the cranial nerves for us to default to our comfort settings.

Television was a slow climb up from the small snippets of the internet, and because shows tend to be shorter than films, they were adequately bite-sized for times when the indica was strong and our interest easily waned. Despite those who protest against the old boob-tube as a "brain drain," there is a compelling layer to the shows we grew up watching that we didn't always catch on our first run.

Pro tip: If you watch anything when you're high, consider using subtitles. While watching at night gives the allure of being in a theatre, if you currently rent a shared space like an apartment, to be a respectful neighbour you can't turn the volume up too loud. It can be hard to follow dialogue when your mind slows down, which makes it easy to fall behind with the story. With subtitles, you get to see the visuals and stay on track with the words if you miss something.

The Simpsons was one of Mike's favourite shows to watch, and as he was perpetually high, I can understand why. Being animated, it has a great mix of colour to keep your focus, and the tongue-in-cheek humour uncovers the writers' brilliance in satire, side-swiping you with comedic irony. I also recommend the American version of *The Office* (already on-point with my awkward sense of humour), which mimics regular working-class lives, imperfect human relationships, and flawed characters—the introspective stoner's cup of tea.

Being in a mental state that reassembles a sponge soaking up experiences, sometimes TV makes it easier to be distracted from our egos and reflect on everyday situations from a broader perspective. I happened to come across an old episode of *The Fresh Prince of Bel-Air* on television one night, post take-out with Jem. By this time, she was curled up in a fetal position on the couch asleep, and I was wide awake finishing off a bag of my dill pickle flavoured potato chips that we got on a snack run a couple days prior. I forget most of the episode, but I do remember singing along–badly–to the show's intro (*Coupla' kids up to no good, started-makin-trouble-in-the-neighbourhood!*) before I got distracted by cat videos on my phone. I tuned in again sometime around the end of the show, when the main character Will (Smith) was in a hotel after pretending to marry a girl so he could have sex with her; she being an old-fashioned "I want to wait until I get married" type.

He and his friend Jazz—an endearing simpleton with a lack of verbal filter—set up a fake wedding. When Will's "wife" is ready to "go all the way," his conscience convinces him to fess up and come clean. The lesson of the episode is painfully refreshing to see in media considering it aired all the way back in 1993, while the #MeToo movement took until 2017 to attract real global attention. Despite the "mature audience" subject rating that is rare for family shows, Will's uncle Phil teaches us that "intimacy requires real commitment," and we all come away a little wiser learning it isn't right to disrespect someone for selfish motives.

In an episode of the show *Community* (an underappreciated little gem), a group of eccentric individuals in a community college arrange a play about drug awareness for a group of children from a visiting middle school. Unfortunately, the role of "drugs" goes to Chevy Chase's character Pierce—the oldest, most crass member with a desire for the spotlight. Dressed as a marijuana leaf, Pierce's love of attention and crude humour inadvertently drives the children to hilariously cheer for drugs. As the group desperately tries to control the damage from the situation, Señor Chang (the school's Asian Spanish teacher) usurps Pierce and goes out on stage:

"Greetings, you little snots!" he says, laughing manically. "Did you expect me to stay the same forever?! I control your lives, and there is nothing you can do!"

As the children riot and start to beat Señor Chang to the ground, the day is saved, and the anti-drug message is reiterated. I loved this episode the first time I watched it, but when I watched it high it was even more of a delight—not because I was smoking pot and watching a man dressed as a marijuana leaf saying he's going to "wear your little brother's skin like pyjamas"—but because I was able to philosophically reflect on the message of the episode. How brilliant it was to see a comical approach to an issue society takes so seriously, without compromising a simple message to warn children about the dangers of drugs. Eccentric adults trying to warn a younger generation about the pitfalls of life exists at the heart of society as we know it today, and although they attempt to teach children how to live, in reality, no one really knows what they're doing.

If you think about it, nothing has really changed.

23
Movies

Getting high before I did something became an appreciation for the act, not something to just pass the time with. Since one of my favourite things to do when I was sober was watch movies, watching them high became my new favourite pastime. Animated films were the best because the bright colours, singing, romance, and drama are everything a psychoactive mind could hope for. Disney movies in particular allowed me to revisit a sense of childlike wonder, and the happy endings were welcomed despite what literature initially influenced them (those Grimm brothers sure did live up to their names). This contrasted my preferred genre in sobriety—horror and thriller movies—which weren't as fulfilling with my high, eagle-like sight that could clearly distinguish the props, CGI, and fake blood; all of it became too distracting after a certain point, which took me out of the experience.

Anything by Tim Burton was a good choice (particularly *The Nightmare before Christmas* and *Edward Scissorhands*), because it dipped into both genres. Not only are his movies cinematically alluring, the characters are engaging, and the soundtracks are downright dreamy thanks to the musical genius of Danny Elfman. Burton often partnered with Johnny Depp in his projects (one of my long-time celebrity obsessions) whose eccentricity fit especially well with Burton's classic fairy tale stories à la "Goth Disney."

Unfortunately, under the intoxication of a high, even when I thought I knew what I wanted to watch, executing my plan became a complicated adventure. On my way to track down my *Wall-E* DVD, I swayed over to the bookshelf where I kept all my movies only to discover that the case in question was empty, and the film was absent—missing in action.

Where else could it be? I wondered, swimming through the murky depths of my mind.

To the laptop! I was probably watching it on my computer last.

When I pressed the button on the side of my computer, I watched the disc tray pop out to reveal a different DVD movie. My unconscious mind fed me the line:

This is not the droid you are looking for.
Well, shit.

I began a hunt from the past, following clues a more sober self had left for me to discover. Suddenly, grasping at past memories about something trivial was now something so crucial to life. As I tried to retrace my steps, Kitkat walked peevishly ahead of me only to stop suddenly, spreading her body out to halt my progress and divert me elsewhere. I translated:

Forget the movie. You belong to me.

It took me a few precious moments to remember what I'd been looking for (although it could have been an hour for all I knew), but I just couldn't remember. Eventually, I decided to pick a different film.

Travelling back to my movie shelf, I stared at the titles long enough to trigger a war between my desire for control and my desire for functionality. Despite my penchant for organizing the titles alphabetically, I was distracted by the weight distribution on the shelves' levels, and moved things around until none of it made sense. Finally, I decided to put aside my neurosis to focus on my propensity for nostalgia, knowing that's what would ultimately lead me here in the future. I picked movies based off of the feelings associated with their memories, and effectively reorganized my collection to be both structurally sound and high-functioning (*Ba-dum-tsss*).

When I watched all my favourite flicks again when I was high, it felt like I was watching them for the first time. It was like visiting with an old friend and catching up with them years later; their story was familiar but I had changed to see them differently, and I couldn't help but smile, laugh, or cry at the nostalgia it evoked within me. With the nostalgic bleeding of my senses, moments in my reality reflected moments of fantasy worlds from the silver screen. My mind shamelessly confused my consciousness to the point where everything became theatrical, and my present experiences merged with fictional ones.

A winged creature fluttered in from the west one night, startling Jem and I as it perched on the armrest of her chair. Defensive from the strangeness of the beast, Jem clutched the lighter in her hand tighter, transforming into Lt. Ellen Ripley with her flamethrower before my eyes. She approached the alien carefully with her weapon, and ignited its flame once she was close to creature's wings. She stayed far enough away that it wouldn't touch, but close enough that it would feel the heat of her warning.

With the arrival of the warmer weather, moths had flocked to the beacon of light from our apartment during the night, but this one was the largest we'd seen. It had to be dealt with like all the rest: chased away with a story to warn its brethren, letting them know they were not welcome in these parts. As Jem's flame inched closer, the creature flapped its grotesque wings and suddenly flew over above us, tapping Jem on her nose in the process.

BOOP!

In the resulting flurry of squeals, it flew back to its perch on the window beside her. Gloating.

Quickly recovering, Jem flashed a look of cold vengeance, the likes of which I had never seen. Taking a cigarette box from nearby, she raised it over her shoulder and rushed forward with deadly precision to ensnare the bug. After removing the small carton from the windowsill with its prize, she sat in contemplation of letting the creature suffer through asphyxiation, or putting it out of its misery with a quick death. Despite her imperative for vengeance, she decided on mercy and let it go. She is a just god.

I craved the intensity of these moments, consuming the escape from reality at any cost. Like the six-fingered man in *The Princess Bride* who screamed at Prince Humperdinck when he raised the dial on the torture device:

"Not to fifty!"

Yes. To fifty I shall go.

High-ho, high-ho.

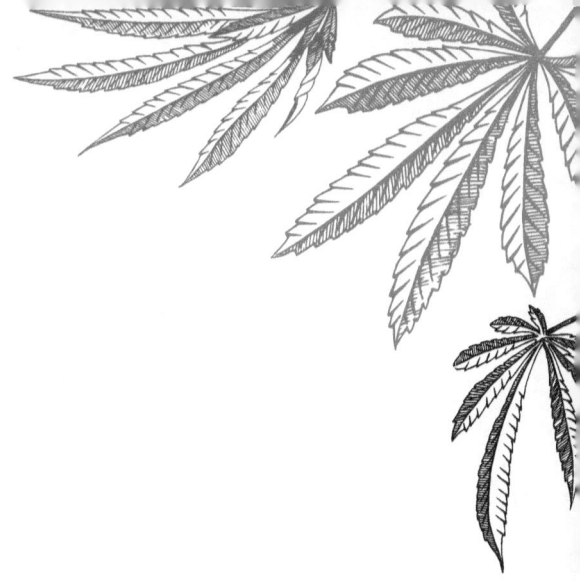

PART V:
BUD-DISM

24
A Matter of Perspective

We are aware of the concept of time as we live, having to plan our daily activities around the number of hours in a day and what we need to accomplish within those hours. But have you ever really stopped to experience the passage of time? When you're high, time perception is altered in a way that concurrently slows down and speeds up any feelings, thoughts, or experiences, which can be both frustrating and exhilarating. This is part of its seduction: a dial gets turned down, and although our physical bandwidth decreases, the mind cranks the senses to eleven. Memories were timelessly compounded for me, and I experienced every minute and every hour simultaneously to the point that when I looked at the clock, I was surprised by how little time had passed.

When Jem went to her younger brother's birthday party to see the latest *Transformers* movie, she told me it was close to three hours long. We contemplated how movies seem to be getting longer these days, with a focus on more action filler rather than story or true substance.

"It's a good thing you weren't high," I said, rolling my head toward her. "That would have lasted *forever.*"

We imagined how she would have stumbled out of the theatre in a daze, confused by the unfamiliar life outside the movie, with the cars as stationary, lifeless machinery in the parking lot.

"I have lived a hundred lifetimes!" she would scream, like a prophet emerging from a time when machines walked the earth like dinosaurs, battling screw and nail for dominance in an endless battle where Mark Walberg is the saviour of humankind.

Being freed from the unilateral direction of time can be a very promising (albeit risky) condition, and having the ability to live in the present as if there was no past and is no future is a strange type of escapism that seems like it comes straight from science fiction. I suppose the concept of time really *can* border on sci-fi when the mind is enthralled by the imagination. A perfect example of this is the theory of parallel universes, also known as the multiverse.

In this theory, time is infinite, and each choice we make creates a series of branched realities, or parallel lives. Considering all the decisions we make throughout our lives, imagine how many universes exist for each alternate choice. Just think: in some dimension—past, present, or future—there could be a version of you affected by different decisions made at specific junctures in your life. How different would this version be from your life now? We've all imagined these moments, and the possibility of taking the knowledge of what we know now back in time. These types of thought exercises have created a lot of popular media, and dusting them out from the crooks of the human mind is nothing short of inspiring. I figure being high is one extra key to unlocking the creative juices.

Contemplating big picture theories is fun and all, but for me, an awareness of the small things I took for granted on a regular basis was just as mind-altering—like becoming aware of the way your eyes ignore the nose in the middle of your face. While it's easy to focus on the future, where we cast all our hopes and dreams, to live in the present moment was a type of freedom I had never even considered.

25
Bud-dism

Getting high was, and continues to be, a very spiritual experience for me. When my corporeal cravings are no longer the focus, I'm able to live in the present with an awareness that becomes a powerful antidepressant which allows both sides of my brain to reach—outstretched toward one another—and form a state of mind no longer divided by my left and right hemispheres. Thinking and feeling simultaneously, my heart and mind became the very core of my existence, and I began to see how one easily influences the other. I feel like the truest version of myself when I'm high, and I feel free to experience a love and devotion for myself that is always overlooked when I'm sober.

If I was ever stuck in a negative loop, getting high would blissfully distract me by putting things in perspective. I could come home after a stressful day at work, and instead of having a cold beer or a glass of wine like some people, I would smoke a joint and suddenly stop over-analyzing why that lady on the subway gave me a dirty look, and start focusing on the important things in life, like if cursive writing was considered body language. This sort of simplicity allowed me to detach from an obsession with logic and a need for control over my environment in order to feel safe.

In Buddhism, to understand suffering is to become enlightened by the impermanence of reality. In other words, when we acknowledge that we control the rate and degree to which we experience stress, change, and our very physical existence, we can control our narrative. We can become aware of the intricacies of life around us, and understand that it is here, in the present, where happiness can truly be found. Buddhism further suggests that with the concept of karma, our souls are consistently reborn to learn lessons, which aid the growth of our spirit toward nirvana, or a state of total enlightenment. Our thoughts and actions elicit the cause and effect of our destinies, and by understanding how we suffer in this lifetime, we are advancing our soul on its journey into future lifetimes, ever-learning our place in the universe and ever-evolving. A man with an unconventional job once personified this lesson for me.

Entertaining is a competitive business, and as a tourist city, Toronto is an extremely competitive environment. In order to stand out, it's common for individuals to try and develop a lucrative idea that attracts an audience, but quite often you can only work with what you have. This man didn't have much, and decided professional cosplay was his way in.

Cosplay (short for costume play) is when an individual dresses up as a fictional character. Believe it or not, it can be a profitable, and people have been able to create a source of income by constructing different outfits to sell, modelling, or being paid to feature as certain characters at events. Some remain as the same character consistently and milk it for all it's worth (like Elvis impersonators), while others have an array of costumes and characters. This individual—let's call him Marty—fell into the former category, and moonlighted as the same character on street corners for years. Usually drawn to the eccentric, I was attracted to him like a moth to a flame, but it soon become obvious to me that he was quite mentally disturbed.

Marty was obsessed by the attention he got and fixated on the idea of becoming an actor, despite obvious criticism and an unwillingness to adapt. Originally working on Hollywood Boulevard in Los Angeles, he had a routine: standing on the same street corner every summer in the original suit of his character (one that was notorious for costume upgrades), and shouting famous epithets that got old real fast. He never understood why his shtick went nowhere, ultimately placing the blame on his audiences. I practically forced my way into his life—singularly focused as I was by my obsession with him—and between his penchant for trying to force the door open into fame, we smoked weed together. He became very introspective, and talked a lot about his lack of finances and how approaching age thirty, he should find a more stable source of income rather than hiding behind the mask of his character.

When we smoked, Marty was cheerful and considerate. He actually acknowledged me in our conversations, stepping away from his usual self-fixation and uncanny ability to make everything about him. Sometimes, I imagined he would have been perfectly fine talking to a mirror, soothed by the sound of his own voice. I'll admit I didn't offer much in the way of conversation (as you know, I'm not much of a talker), but I was enamoured with his popularity, so I stuck around.

Occasionally he was bolstered by fresh media coverage which, unfortunately, started his madness anew. Ultimately, I grew bored of the increasing desperation in his attempts for attention and his inability to see how predictable he was. It was a very mind-opening experience to see the pattern in his choices—the inability to change and adapt to unfavourable results which continued to surprise and frustrate him—which led me to the conclusion that this karma thing may have something to it, and his soul may be stuck on a particularly poignant life lesson.

I'm quite partial to the idea of a recycled soul journeying through lifetimes and heading toward some end goal. Reincarnation and karma go hand in hand in Buddhism, and the belief is that an individual's actions, good or bad, attract a similar good or bad result. The idea is to refine our thoughts and actions to learn over lifetimes with the ultimate goal of evolving, or "levelling up" to reach a state of self-realization or enlightenment. Cannabis became a spiritual tool for me, and I used it to engage in this kind of self-discovery.

In Eastern religious philosophies, there are energy centres within our physical bodies that make up the spirit, called chakras. There are seven chakras, starting from the root located at the base of our spine. Moving upwards is the sacral chakra (just below the belly button), the solar plexus chakra (in the upper abdomen or stomach area), the heart chakra (in the centre of the chest), the throat chakra, the third eye chakra (in the middle of the forehead or between the eyes), and the crown chakra (at the very top of our heads). They can open (expand) or close (contract) depending on the circumstances of a person's life. I came to learn about these through my deep-dive into occult interests and alternative medicine, including the study of reiki, a Japanese healing modality which involves the manipulation of these energies. These energy centres are responsible for various emotional, mental, and physical abilities of our human spirit, and it's the crown chakra that's responsible for a divine connection that is greater than ourselves. When I talk of my new-found spirituality, I speak of this connection and the ability to open up to that which is all.

When time stood still under the meditation of being high, I was able to sit with my thoughts and explore the interconnected experiences that helped shape me, and my third eye (theorized to increase perception, awareness, and spiritual communication) opened to the world. I imagined a colourful network above my head, the point of origin at the tip of my scalp and extending upwards and outwards like a beacon balancing on top. It's as if this beacon was calling out to a mother ship, and like some alien species, I was telepathically connected to the world, suddenly craving unity. The depth of feeling seemed like more than just my imagination, and sometimes the emotions of others around me became so clear they were palpable; they felt so very like my own thoughts, as if I were the one living with these feelings instead of them. I fast-tracked from sympathy to empathy, as if there was suddenly a collective conscious I was tapping into. My desire to connect with others was so strong, and I wanted to do good in and for humanity, as if my life depended on it. Perhaps it was a glimpse of a purpose.

Unity with others sparked an idea, and sharing became a goal, but the prerequisite work was internal. First, I needed to discover peace, happiness, and contentment within myself.

This is how I became a "Bud-dist."

Bud-dism, or the exploration into my own version of enlightenment, revolves around reflection and determining one's inner growth through self-knowing. Similar to Buddhism in that it holds the same beliefs in the importance of mindfulness, karma, and a focus on presence, Bud-dism is coined after the THC-saturated bud of the cannabis plant.

We know cannabis and its constituents have existed for millennia and fixated as we are in Western society to produce and accumulate, while we were busy taking the plant at face value—deconstructing it into hemp products to create wealth—Eastern societies and Indigenous Peoples saw it for its spiritual potential. History documents cannabis' use as a religious tool, a source of happiness, and perhaps even a gift from the gods. Is it a coincidence that scientists named the receptors in our brains which bind to THC "Anandamide," which comes from the Sanskrit word for bliss? Interestingly, most ancient Buddhist texts are written in Sanskrit.

I imagine Bud-dism as a sect of spirituality that uses cannabis as a tool to unlock the greater mysteries of the universe. To do this, contemplation is necessary for self-actualization, and THC greatly enhances our ability to contemplate. The more we deconstruct our personal experiences at the depth of our psyches, the more we can realize we are all souls having a human experience. All of us are a part of this experience, and although our exact circumstances differ, our perceptions are rooted in the same psychological phenomenon we still study to this day.

As a Bud-dist, I believe our lives play out in cycles and without knowing it, we face the same problems over and over again like Marty, until some lesson is learned and we intrinsically progress forward—this is the idea behind Buddhist karma. The Bud-dist has a tool (cannabis) to challenge their thoughts and beliefs, seeing things simply as they present themselves, objectively, with emotions acknowledged but separate. Seeing this truth allows one to re-learn about themselves, creating space for the person they want to be. You could say it all comes down to brain chemistry, but what are we if not our brains? The cannabis connection unlocks a part of us—one that is familiar but foreign—under the harsh light of the reality we have been living. Recognizing where the mind and body synchronize or diverge offers an awareness of self we aren't always privileged to notice.

26
Writing To Purge

When I first began smoking cannabis, experiences came hard and fast in ways I couldn't comprehend, but the more I tried it, the easier it was to recognize the value of a high. Reflective thought soon became unavoidable, and along with an awareness of the many intricacies of being stoned, there also came a series of revelations. These experiences were so new and overwhelming to me that mere introspection evolved into challenges of my morals and beliefs. My biased opinions of people who smoked were the first to relent. Next, I developed a need to connect to others and express the feelings within me that I tried so hard to stifle all my life.

When I was high, I felt pulled to others, as if by an invisible thread, and had a sense of kinship. I had a few close friends, but I always felt I was holding a part of myself back from them. Jem was really the only exception, but her presence in my life up until now ebbed and flowed like the change of the tides. Silence was the by-product of the solitude I found comfort in, but under the haze of a high, these new feelings were persistent and eager to knock down the walls I had built around myself. They floated around in my brain like the microscopic fibres that shadow our retinas as we age: difficult to focus on, despite their obvious presence, and yet impossible to ignore.

The problem was that so far in my life, any opportunity to form my thoughts into words and express them in the real world fell short of my expectations, often resulting in personal embarrassment. I could live with my own judgement, but I feared the thoughts of others about me. Just like the French paper brought to the principal's office, I sabotaged my own cries for help because I was uncomfortable with the attention it brought—but without asking for it, I could never receive it. I neglected to use my voice for expression when I was younger, and as a result I was never able to develop it. Despite this, my thoughts never stopped.

Writing is a cathartic experience for the introvert. Being far from charismatic, I found that writing seemed like the only way for me to communicate appropriately since I could take time to think, pick out the right words to accurately describe my thoughts, and physically purge them from my head. This didn't change when I was stoned, although the thoughts became more relentless than usual, and it wasn't long until I needed to put them somewhere.

I never planned to write about my experience, it just so happened that once I started smoking I felt compelled to. It was like squeezing the pus out of a festering wound so it could build new, healthy tissue. Thoughts and connections bubbled up and rose into my brain, and I felt the words creeping up my gullet in a way that made me feel I needed to vomit and purge them. Our bodies are pretty good at knowing what they need, and sometimes all we can do is just go along with it, trusting in the human hardwiring for survival. You know how vomiting when you feel sick makes you feel better? Well, I hope you're wearing protection, because what you have in your hands is the physical representation of my brain vomit. And boy, does it feel good to get it out.

I'm a firm believer in everything happening for a reason. Before moving in with Jem and my exploration with cannabis, I received a journal as a Christmas present from a high school friend. A few years earlier, I had a conversation with this friend about her concern for her significant other and his indulgence in weed. I didn't know what to say to ease her mind, and I was ashamed to admit to my initial disgust and the defensive feeling of elitism it triggered in me. The journal she gave me was a shimmering forest-green, covered in leaves that were outlined in gold from front to back along its smooth surface. At the time I got it, I didn't know it would become the reshaped landscape of my own psychoactive mind, and guide my emotions—raw and open—into a present that wasn't yet fully realized.

I began to write my experiences and thoughts down while high, and it wasn't long before I found them becoming more profound, and even kind of funny. My first pearl of "weedsdom" was particularly insightful:

I think they should legalize weed and use it to punish criminals by making them think really hard about what they've done.

Owing to the fact that your brain is in overdrive, being locked in a cell with nothing but thoughts of your crimes was, what I thought, an effective form of rehabilitation, à la *A Clockwork Orange*.

Originally, it was my intention to collect these thoughts for casual self-indulgence and a fun pick-me-up if needed because, yes, I do laugh at my own jokes (I consider it a superpower). I struggled with the idea that perhaps something so personal could become meaningful to others, but eventually it grew beyond myself. I am unavoidably the pro-tagonist of this memoir, but it was never my intention to assume this role, as it was merely to share with others, and I dread coming across as pretentious.

One of the great battles I faced as I attempted to write was the speed of my mind against the sedated movements of my body. While I was high, I couldn't write as fast as my thoughts came to me, which I found odd, considering the way time seems to slow down when you are intoxicated. If I could have articulated my experience to you through a musical, I certainly would have! It felt like one in my head.

Unsurprisingly, there are a few problems with trying to write a book about smoking weed, the foremost being ambiguity. How can you intel-ligently describe an experience that is subjective? Despite common physical effects, there is no way my narrative can be representative of all individuals. It's like taking a picture on vacation only to discover that when you show it to others, you weren't able to accurately capture the beauty of what you saw with your own eyes. I felt that way about a cake once, and it was a damned shame I couldn't share it with someone.

A second problem is logistics. High thoughts are very much like golden snitches from the world of *Harry Potter*: hard to catch and hold on to, but if you can, each one is a winner. Since my thoughts were going a mile a minute, it was a struggle to transcribe them onto paper before they were lost. I did find that these thoughts never quite disappeared though, and if I focused hard enough, I could recover them within a certain time by picking up the threads that lingered and pulling myself back into that specific mindset long enough to write them down. Pinning down the words established a save point where I could pick up from, and if I didn't, I feared they would be lost forever. It makes sense how weed makes certain people tired; it's exhausting to chase all the buzzing thoughts in your head when they go in whatever direction they want.

A third problem when writing about smoking weed, and perhaps the most important, is discernment. When I first started putting ideas together, I wrote down everything that I thought was interesting when I was high, only later to discover that I think *everything* is interesting when I'm high. (This too, I found interesting.)

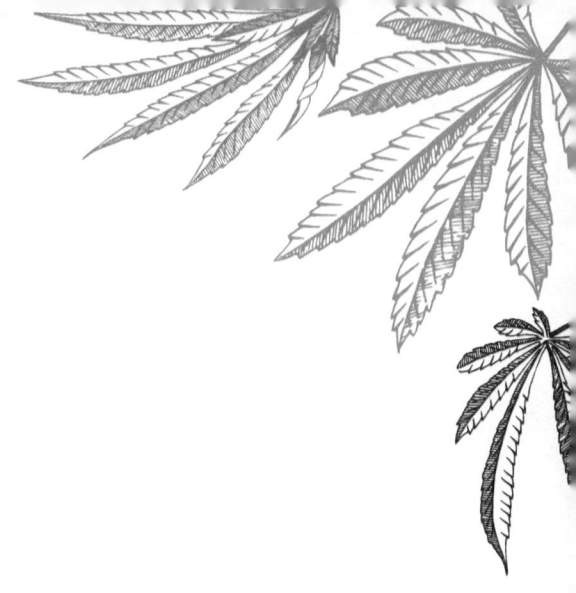

PART VI:
SECOND SIGHT

27
Tourism

It's often said that the eyes are a window to the soul, and since they play such a huge role in processing stimuli, the amount of light around you can affect the kind of high you experience. Light plays a role in keeping us awake and engaged, affecting neurotransmitters in our brain which control our sleep-wake cycles. Many people use cannabis products to help their insomnia, and it's true that eyelids tend to become heavy in the low part of a high, making it easier to succumb to sleep in the darkness. Other times, cannabis can be stimulating.

I've come to terms with the fact that I will never be a "morning person," considering my tendency to self-sabotage and snooze my alarms for thirty minutes (I even set my alarms for work considering the amount of snooze I can get away with before needing to get out of bed), so it was strange to feel productive when I got high during the day. I appreciated the nice little jolt of happy hormones that I felt when the light stimulated my brain, which gave me the little push I needed to follow through and accomplish something.

That being said, a day-high (cannabis indulgence anytime the sun is up), although similar to its famous cousin the "wake and bake" (indulging immediately after waking up in the morning), is markedly different.

I once chose to partake in the ritual of the wake and bake (for science!), but was quickly dissuaded by the handicapping result it had on me. Getting high as soon as I woke up, I experienced the opposite of the productive feeling I had during my other day-highs; even with the sunlight shining, I could do no more than stick to the couch in helplessness and ruminate. Still sluggish from a recent awakening, the effects of the weed nailed me into the ground like a tent, as a physical representation of "bleh." I think my issue was that, again, I was putting too much expectation onto an experience . . . that, or I chose my strain incorrectly: sativa would be more likely to stimulate my mind, while indica was more likely to physically ground me. There's always a learning curve to adapt to, and practice makes perfect.

While I found the wake and bake wasn't for me, the effect of the sunlight and some good company was. Hanging out with Adam, Jem, and Connor (one of Jem's old friends from high school) one day, we were discussing Canadian norms, growing up in the nineties, and our mutual love of coffee when the munchies kicked in. I didn't feel prepared to face the world outside of our safe space in the apartment, but the collective need for food triggered the equally primitive herd mentality to seek it, so we decided to go on a food run. We left the apartment and walked down the hall, pressing the button to summon the elevator which would take us down to the main floor. Distracted by the full length mirrors beside the doors, I looked at myself, conscious of the mismatched sweatpants and obscene T-shirt I was wearing. Thankfully, I did not give a fuck.

When the elevator doors chimed and opened, we all looked in at the petite raven-haired woman with her dog who had arrived to share the elevator. Even at the best of times, I'm unable to stifle my squeals of delight at an animal, and I was certainly not at my best.

"Doggy!" my voice squeaked traitorously as we all piled in.

The dog's ears raised slightly, and it tilted its head at me in curiosity. The woman pulled its' leash closer to her torso.

Out of our minds, all four of us rode the elevator down staring intently at this dog, simultaneously oblivious and awkwardly aware of the woman's presence next to it. In the resulting silence, I felt like I could sense the collective thoughts around me, noting that some of us seemed more embarrassingly aware of our inebriated state than others. With my paranoia in full swing, I couldn't decide whether to stay quiet or engage in conversation. A troubled childhood made Adam free from the fear of what others thought, so he spoke up.

"How old is he or she?" Adam asked casually. Having worked at a kennel for years, he was unabashedly curious and a dog lover.

Mumble mumble said the woman.

I only heard the sounds as a response, but I could tell she wasn't interested in conversation. I screeched at Adam in my mind:

Traitor! You'll out us!

He continued a superficial conversation with the woman while I begin counting the number of floors until our escape. One painful stop at a time, I wondered what the first clue she would pick up on would be. A whiff of smoke clinging to our clothes? Our red, tired eyes? The slight sway of our bodies as we adjusted to the elevators' movement?

"That dog has a great personality," Adam was saying.

PING!

Time to make our escape!

Don't run, dogs can sense fear.

After we all shuffled out of the elevator, I walked as fast as I could into freedom and fresh air to get away from my anxiety and discomfort. The others followed, and Adam brought up the rear, sauntering in his familiar carefree way.

The sunshine was glorious in the mellow warmth of the summer, and its brightness sent a jolt of electricity through my mind, resetting the synapses as we walked across a residential street and through a popular alleyway behind some shops. We spied a McDonald's close by, and the golden "M" beckons even the most lethargic of stoners with its promise of salt, fat, and ice-creamy goodness. We entered the restaurant and stood at the back of the crowd, staring at the menu like pirates looking for lost treasure, our mouths agape in possibility.

There were two adorable teens behind the counter: young girls in their uniforms and shiny name tags hurriedly processing orders. While waiting in line, I decided to give them backstories:

Katerina and Nicole were good friends since they met early in high school, both a part of the volleyball team at *random location*. Nicole's parents were both lawyers and although well off, wanted their only daughter to learn the value of hard work, insisting that she pay for half of her schooling. She wanted to be a make-up artist, and despite her parent's attempt to dissuade her to go to school for "a real job," they eventually came to terms with her determination by imposing limits.

Katerina's goal in life was much shorter sighted: she was working toward a car. Knowing her friend already worked at the McDonald's close to her house, Katerina begged Nicole to petition her McBoss to hire her. One day both the girls were working a particularly busy shift at work. Katerina had been at the cash register for what seemed like hours as the steady stream of customers flowed through the doors of the small restaurant, while Nicole worked tirelessly behind the counter dropping fries and nuggets, spinning iced coffees, and getting her swirls just right on the soft-serve machine.

"Can I help who's next?" Katerina called out to get Adam's attention, him being next in line, and the most visible among the crowd.

He was the tallest of our group of four—skinny in a sleeveless striped shirt with a grizzly beard and a bald head which was clearly shaved to camouflage his premature baldness.

"Uh, yeah," he said, taking two large steps toward her.

"Can I get two Big Macs with large fries, an apple strudel, a carrot muffin, a Smarties McFlurry . . . snack size . . ."

He paused, squinting his eyes at the all-day breakfast menu on the right as Katerina hurriedly located the buttons on the register to key in his order. She waited a few seconds, glancing up at him before asking if he wanted anything else. He blinked once slowly and turned his head to face her.

"I only want one hash brown, but I know they usually come with two. Can I just get one?"

"Um, just a second let me ask," she replied, turning over her shoulder to see Nicole behind her with her eyebrows slightly raised as if to say, "I guess?" or "Is this guy for real?"

Katerina turned back to him.

"Sure, that's ok. That will be $18.35."

"Sweet," he said, smiling.

He stood there for a few seconds before muttering and patting his pockets. He finally pulled out his wallet and handed her a twenty-dollar bill. She opened the register and rifled out his change before grabbing the receipt and a pen to write.

"What's the name for the order?" she asked.

"Alevein," he said.

She hovered the pen over the receipt as her brain tried to process what she heard.

". . . How do you spell that?" she finally managed to say, hearing a barely perceived snort coming from behind to her.

"A . . . l . . . e . . . v . . . i . . . e . . . n," he said slowly, clearly making it up along the way.

Katerina shot a quick glance behind him to me. My eyebrows rose as my eyes widened in embarrassment, and I tried focusing them on the counter in front of me to maintain my innocence through stillness.

Katerina spelled out the letters and looked at Adam, trying to make sense of how to pronounce their random compilation. By now a couple of extra staff members were coming from the back as reinforcements for the ever-growing stream of customers, and she had to shake her confusion away so she could keep the line going. The other orders from our group were easy enough, and were processed quicker as a result.

When the food was ready, Nicole and a young recruit from the kitchen (who I named Hussein) began handing over the orders. One by one the names were called out and people reached eagerly over the counter for their bags. Out of the corner of her eye, Katerina could see Hussein and Nicole scanning the strange name spelled out on the top of one of the receipts, pausing with unknown expressions on their faces before ignoring it to reach for another. Soon the time came when it couldn't be ignored, and it was Hussein who reluctantly picked up the slip.

"Al-eve-ien?" he said sheepishly in his thick European accent, before looking around to see a response.

Katerina looked at my brother as we all stood together, each holding a take-out bag with our food waiting patiently (except for Jem who was lost to the salty lure of her fries). He was staring up at the menu again, oblivious to the name called. Hussein leaned over to Katerina

"How do you pronounce this?" he asked.

Nicole came up from behind them and they all hovered around the strange name, silent and unsure of what they were looking at. Katerina spoke up after a few moments of silence. She didn't know how to pronounce it either, but at least she knew who it belonged to.

"Al-evian?" her voice was small and timid as she looked into the crowd. I subtly elbowed Adam out of his trance, and he looked around, oblivious, until he spotted the three teens behind the counter looking at him expectantly.

"Oh! That's me!" he said, taking the bag.

We walked out together, each holding our prize. Once we were gone, Katerina felt Nicole lean in to whisper softly into her ear.

"That guy was full of shit," she said, a smug smile playing at the corner of her lips before she turned back to the fryer.

Outside, I turned to my brother. "You're full of shit" I said as he unwrapped the first of his two burgers, his eyes were wide with amusement.

"Almost gave them my name. Tried to get creative at the last minute. I just went with it."

As I discovered that day, when one chooses to get high during the day, they are making both a statement and a decision: that they allow the possibility of people seeing them act like a total idiot, and that they are OK with it. The paranoia of a high exacerbates when reflecting on the difficulty of tasks that, under sobriety, are usually simple, but it's true that we grow most by triumphing over challenges. Becoming comfortable with my discomfort was something I was acclimatizing to, and I found the choice to forge ahead without fear of judgement filled me with the thrill of discovery and an ever-expanding sense of freedom.

28
High In The City

I was experiencing a time of exploration in my life, one that took me back to that same feeling of riding my bike down a newly discovered street at my dad's house. I felt a similar sense of liberation by exploring the nuances of my mind and rewriting my experiences of isolation from the inside out. I got out more from the smoky den in the bachelorette pad I shared with Jem, and felt passably comfortable about behaving myself in a crowd of people. As I became confident enough in my skills to pass as sober, my desire for adventure became overwhelming. I wanted to see how I would experience familiar situations under the influence.

Although I've lived around Toronto all my life, I had never taken the time to experience or appreciate it. With the power of flower I was emboldened, and I booked a week off work to dedicate time to exploring my outside surroundings with new eyes. The city is similar to a space port in a science fiction movie in that people of different ethnicities and walks of life from all over the world congregate. The environment can be hostile and unpredictable, but like anywhere, if you keep your head down and your wits about you, you won't run into much trouble. For better or for worse, people tend to mind their own business.

The diversity makes the landscape compelling, and pockets of culture compete for space at the heart of the city. A short walk is all it takes to discover neighbourhoods nestled away from the busy streets with Victorian style houses meticulously maintained and hidden among the trees. The core of downtown is the complete opposite, studded with commercial districts and tall skyscrapers, high-priced ad space, pollution, and crowds of people that barely pay attention to where they are going. There's a little bit of everything in Toronto, from the rocky spits of land that join with Lake Ontario (which we generously call beaches), to developing real estate plots that look like they belong in a post-apocalyptic environment with their dull greys and crumbling exteriors. Growing up as a pedestrian in the city I loved its diversity, but once I started driving it became a nightmare to navigate.

Toronto is home to the CN Tower—one of the most iconic tourist attractions in the world—and even though I had lived in the city for decades, I had never been there. To me, the idea of paying to ride an elevator up hundreds of metres to look down at a glass floor and then go back down didn't sound like the most exciting thing in the world.

But what about being high up *and* high? I never considered myself to be afraid of heights, but who knew what was possible with my primal instincts left permission to roam. I decided to bring my one-hitter and see how bold I felt when I got there.

Who would have thought there would be a security check before going up?

Joining the line to the elevators with my fellow tourists, the sight of security and the metal detectors stopped me in my tracks. As I clutched my purse closer to protect my sacred stash hidden within, I couldn't help the flood of thoughts going through my mind, which mingled with the paranoia from the THC I ingested before entering.

Oh-my-God-I'm-not-going-to-go-to-jail-for-this-shit!

Luckily, I don't look threatening or suspicious, and I'm really good at playing dumb. I pretended to look in my purse, wandering off slowly toward a nearby vending machine to give myself time to think. I passed a floating shelf on the wall and spied an opportune corner between the machine and a metal bar running along the floor to casually place my suspicious package (aka one-hitter). I hoped it would still be there when I got back down, and that I wouldn't be pulled aside on my way out with:

"Ma'am I'm going to need you to come with me . . ."

It was a small sacrifice leaving it behind, but recreational marijuana wasn't legal at this time, and I needed to consider the weight of choosing a life of crime.

This fucking tower better be worth it.

The view was indeed incredible; the city below looked like a computer circuit with the alternating heights of buildings and different shimmering colours. The cars on the roadways below looked like slow-travelling dust mites. I felt like I was high up in a birdcage, surrounded by metal bars that destroyed any pretense of freedom by whispering "you can look but don't touch." For an extra twelve dollars (an obscene amount of money to spend to advance an extra 100 feet) I waited a ridiculously long amount of time for another elevator to bring me to a smaller, more vacant platform that resembled a bunker, which offered another view. I gave it a solid "meh" before recalling the elevator.

I figured I spent about an hour up in the tower, weaving between bodies of tourists taking pictures from a section of glass flooring and reading historical facts from the walls. When I returned to the ground, I casually employed the same purse-searching technique to lead me to where I had left my precious package, and was ecstatic to find it was still there. God bless that I wasn't in the militant United States of America.

Even still, my paranoid mind contrived the idea that a guilty party would flee the scene quickly, so I tried to take my sweet-ass time lingering. Putting on a good show of "oooh's" and "ahhs," I furrowed my brows in concentration as I meandered through the gift shop. I even stuck around to watch a short film on the history of the Toronto Transit Commission (TTC) before finally departing. It was mildly interesting, but overall a waste of time.

Alas, I must suffer for my art.

My next stop was a castle: Casa Loma. Located in a nostalgic neigh-bourhood, I had visited this popular tourist attraction numerous times in my past and absolutely loved it. This particular city landmark, now a museum, was originally constructed in 1914 and was once the largest private residence in Canada. It was like stepping into a live-action version of the board game *Clue*; it boasted a library, a conservatory, a billiards room, stables, and a never completed pool. Just like I'd always imagined a good castle to have, there were even small, narrow staircases concealed into the walls that acted as secret passageways to various parts of the castle. Under the influence, it seemed like a perfect place to explore, and I was excited for my psychoactive mind to play.

I took a short bus ride, emerging from the tunnels of Dupont to the bottom of Spadina, finally climbing a hill to reach the looming structure sitting behind its stone walls. I decided the distance was just enough that I could get a couple good tokes in, allowing the THC just enough time to penetrate my cells before I arrived at the entrance.

As I approached the courtyard, ready to blaze, I took out my Bic lighter and flicked it. The small wheel spun uselessly, igniting a flame that died instantly.

click click

....

CLICK CLICK CLICK

....

Nothing. And wouldn't you know it, castles don't sell lighters. There were no convenience stores in the area either.

Well, shit.

My plans fizzled out as efficiently as my cheap, dollar store lighter. I already had my day planned, and since I didn't have a car to drive, I sure as hell wasn't going to travel back home by bus defeated. I stood swearing on the sidewalk, mid-ascension to my goal and angry at my luck. It was a gorgeous summer day and the sun was bright and hot as it winked through the trees around me. The birds were shrill in my ears, and after I finished seething, I tried to reason with myself. I *had* already bought my admission ticket, and I was quite literally steps away from the destination, so I decided to continue on. Thankfully, the idea of exploring a castle never loses its appeal.

In retrospect, I'm glad I wasn't high. I fixated on the steep winding staircases, secret passages, and tripping hazards, reflecting that I probably would have gotten myself killed. One missed step with my fucked senses and me and the other tourists would have collided, falling down the old architecture like human dominoes.

So far, my batting average was a disappointing 0-2, having failed to secure a memorable high for both of my city attractions. I decided my last destination would be a place that never failed to sustain my interest: The Toronto Zoo.

It was a trip down memory lane in more ways than one. I took a bus to the outskirts of the city in Scarborough, where I grew up, and where the zoo was built away from the majority of human congestion. The parking lot was more crowded than I anticipated even though it was a weekday, and there were more families with children than I had hoped for. I didn't care too much, I was there to see animals after all, and humans are just a different sort I was prepared to also observe.

Once I stepped off the bus and the gates were in view, I was faced with my first problem. Where does one light up a prohibited substance when surrounded by witnesses? The parking lot on the way to the entrance gates provided sufficient cover, and I rationalized that since smokers are notorious for their callous lighting up wherever they are, I would blend in pretty easily. By the time someone smelled what was going on, I would be long gone.

The smoke hit my bloodstream quickly like usual, and with my one-hitter I was able to look like I was smoking a (perfectly legal) cigarette. A couple puffs was all it took before I was on my way.

One ticket to the animal kingdom, please. I hear the call of my people.

Even though I picked up a map, I followed my feet. It was another perfect summer day in the city with wide blue skies, spotlights of heat, and gentle breezes to cool the skin. All the greenery set the scene on my walk through nature with Mother Earth. Like most zoos, this one was divided into pavilions of the world where animals are similarly located: Europe and Asia, Indonesia, Malasia, Africa, North America, the Tundras. Each area was designed to mimic stepping into the world of these animals, trying to make up for the fact that they are behind cages and windows. Around the animals are usually boards with information about them, detailing their origins, behaviours, and breeding patterns—very interesting stuff. I usually liked to read them, but the buzzing of my senses distracted me too easily. My brain would absorb the words, but their meanings wouldn't register, so I found myself reading the same sentence over and over again.

Then I got lost, and I couldn't figure out how to read the map.

Devolved with the memory of a goldfish, I circled the domains, continuously trying to use the so-called shortcuts that the map boasted. I felt the pull of something, perhaps the unconscious threads of past experience, but I ended up going nowhere. I moved through the stages of grief, past anger and denial toward acceptance, where I eventually decided to drop the pretense of being in control. I resigned myself to once again let my feet steer.

I snuck another toke down the dirt path of the Aboriginal trails, which are conveniently ignored by tourists (much like our ugly involvement with their history). Sidetracked by a nest of clovers on my way out, I spent the next ten minutes searching for a four-leaf clover despite the inquisitive gazes of the occasional passerby.

An awkward interaction with a child and her grandparents reminded me that it was best to avoid interacting with all animals whether they were segregated by obvious confinements or not. The kid was standing up on a small ledge facing a tank of otters (AKA snake mammals that slither back in forth in water). Whenever one would swim by the glass she screamed, and with my highly responsive senses, I flinched at the shrill sound. When the grandmother made eye contact with me, she smiled sheepishly.

Shit. Shit. How does social interaction work again? Oh yes! Establish common ground!

"Quite a set of lungs on that one!" I said.
It was all I could think of.

Oh dear, now she looks self-conscious. Maybe she feels like she needs to apologize, but she shouldn't have to because kids will be kids and this is Grandma's special girl . . .

In the future, it would probably be best if I had a chaperone.

Like my imprisoned kin, I acted on instinct. My thoughts processed the visual input immediately, focusing on the key messages:
I had a giggle at the trash panda (commonly known as a racoon), in his enclosure. We both knew he was there because he wanted to be, able to escape at any time with those dexterous paws.
Lynx cats must have been at the top tier of feline worship for the ancient Egyptians; their pointy ear tufts signal distinction, and the sharp black outlines around their eyes, combined with the smoothly pointed furry jowls, look just like the decorated visages of Pharaohs. Did you know the ancient Egyptian word for cat is "mau"? It's only a slight tweak to "meow."
If I hadn't been tripped-out already, the movements of the octopus would have made me so. There was obvious strength in those arms and watching them curl upon themselves reminded me of the demon tree from the movie *Evil Dead*. If those tendrils caught you in their grasp, you'd be powerless against them, mostly because there are fucking EIGHT of them.

What if the tentacles were like Hydra heads that grew back in pairs when you cut them off . . .

There's a reason that penguins are so popular. Nestled in the shade under a canopy in the penguin-viewing area, when it's showtime, the birds know it. Walking out together like a mob, the birds arrive dressed in their finest. Except for a little fluffy one trailing behind, the five of them were a social clique, fitting nicely into the human role.

Smile for the cameras boys, smile and wave.

They all performed their tricks, diving in the water and jumping for treats in perfect synchronized fashion—they knew the drill. Despite the show, all I could seem to focus on was the fluffy one, so obviously segregated from the group and with a green poop stain on his feathers. Every so often he got close to the others and they took turns chasing him away as if to say, "Get out of here kid, this is grown-up work."

All of this was highly entertaining to my distorted mind, and human and animal characteristics clashed endlessly throughout the day: I learned Pelicans basically dismantle their throats to eat. Spider monkeys do look like spiders (good job, taxonomist), and Pokémon are real (*Who's that Pokémon? It's Mudkip! He's an Axolotl!*). Although gorillas are scary, they are indeed our distant ancestors—both types of mothers can breastfeed and break up fights at the same time.

The most interesting creatures at the zoo that day were the lone photographers who curiously populated each animal zone. Although they were in close proximity to one another, their body language indicated they were not together. Their plumage was similar: safari hat, tinted sunglasses, a vest and backpack. They all wore a strap around their necks, and held the camera it attached to firmly with both hands. The device clicked enthusiastically at every minute movement that was made by their animal subject, and every time one of them snapped a picture, they all seemed to snap together.

"Oh my God, the glare is too bright," one said from beside me.

Sitting in a wheelchair, he spoke to no one in particular. I was happy to note that this was an inclusive species; ableism had no home here.

The sighting of this camera-wielding creature amused me. What is their purpose? Are they taking pictures for a magazine or to build their portfolios? Or are they here for pleasure, taking pictures for the simple purpose of something to show to others?

The social media bandwagon confuses me at the best of times, and when it comes to over-sharing, taking pictures of the commonalities of life screams:

"Look at this picture of what I'm eating!" VALIDATE MEEEE.

I spiralled into further drug-fueled existentialist thought: how many of the pictures we take do we actually look at again? In my mind, we take pictures to remember something, but you will never be on your death bed wanting to see the picture of a salad you ate when you were twenty-five. Is this born from a fear of memory failure, or to provide proof to outsiders that your experiences are valid?

As social creatures we share to connect—we crave companionship and interaction—whether we like it or not. We have a need to communicate our thoughts and feelings, consciously or otherwise. At the very least, sometimes all we want is the presence of another, to share the same space. In the absence of this, there is loneliness. Perhaps loneliness is driven by fear of sharing and being rejected, which results in a self-fulfilling prophecy that makes us keep to ourselves (I know this was my reality when I was younger, finding my way after my parent's separation).

Regardless, one thing that I've come to believe from my experience with cannabis is that despite our evolution as a species, the need to share is so deep, it's practically embedded in our cells. Biologically speaking, we have a genetic desire to reproduce by sharing and propagating our DNA. Sometimes, our needs are so primitive it's easy to regress on the quest to pursue them.

29
Animal Planet

It's not my intention to offend, but if you are uncomfortable with the notion of being compared to an animal, if you have an ego that insists you are "big-boned" rather than fat, or if you have terrible sense of humour, I would recommend reading no further (although if you made it this far I would be shocked).

In a world with technological advances like ours, sometimes it's hard to imagine that when it comes down to it, we are just damned, dirty apes. We are bipedal, mostly hairless mammals that still act (and sometimes look) like a bunch of animals in a modernized jungle. Generally the delineation is solid, but sometimes it's fun to watch the lines blur. As a species we are still learning, and it's almost as if we've advanced so far that our DNA doesn't know how to deal with where we find ourselves in the world we've created. Somewhere along the evolutionary train we inherited these big, beautiful brains, but even after all these millennia, we've complicated things and forget that we are still a part of nature.

That we are all animals of this planet is blatantly obvious through the haze of a high, when our perceptions of people and situations shift. Cannabis peels back our human narcissism and egocentrism to show us our origins, where our primal need for survival and acceptance are laid bare. Psychedelics penetrate the grey matter of our being—past all the pomp and circumstance surrounding us—and triggers the ancestral knowledge in our brain. The green urges us to go, and we are all organic machinery in action.

If you isolate the experience from a bigger picture, perhaps human beings aren't all that complicated. Our existence becomes complicated through our socialization into the collective, because at the top of the food chain, there isn't much to hold us accountable to one another unless we create rules. Trying to discover where and how we fit in, and battling with inner demons that make us feel separate and alone is something we all face. As a social species, we crave connection, love, and acceptance. Although we shouldn't define our worth through others, our connections can define us. All of this is most evident when it comes to our intimate relationships, especially those involving the search for a mate.

Generally being a monogamous species, we have an almost animal-istic desire to mate, and whatever that mate looks like—in terms of gender or sexuality—is a moot point because anything goes. A quick side note here for those triggered by this statement in case you didn't heed my earlier warning: Whatever exists is natural, because nature *is* existence. Existence is a product of survival, and it doesn't matter what you believe in because it doesn't change the way things exist. Animals in the wild could give two shits about whether a male seahorse gives birth instead of the traditional female; they survive because they know how to mind their own business.

Remember Simba, we must all take our place in the circle of life.

I first started to notice our connection to the animal kingdom while watching the interactions of my kin from a streetcar window, as it slowly made its way through the crowded city streets one evening. True to the nature of a psychedelic mind, I had a revelation that a guy brave enough to approach a female horde (in clubs, events, various social settings of young'uns) is the equivalent to the sperm that braves the hostile envi-ronment of the uterus to reach the egg. Fortune does indeed favour the bold, and it's these raw behaviours, which are driven by our primitive desires, that are practically translucent in the haze of a high.

Expanding my perspective made me feel like I was aging backwards. Growing up as a stodgy, annoyingly-mature child, it wasn't until I reached my late twenties that I became interested in the idea of taking life less seriously and going to clubs to dance, drink, and fool around. By this time, most of my friends had grown out of this stage just as I was learning to embrace it. Luckily Jem, my go-to gal, was usually up for a night out, even when it was just to humour me because she was no longer on the prowl. Bless her heart.

Growing up is realizing that men and women are perpetually out of sync with one another. As females, we generally look for security because of our historical lack of power. Men, driven by the pull of their hormones and a need to propagate, are led by sex. I always thought it would be funny to shed humour on this awkward truth by interrupting a porno with footage of a baby crying and watch the cognitive dissonance ensue.

Just as the animals do, we seek out mates with distinguishing features through sexual dimorphism to unconsciously propagate the species. Going out was a mating game, and I played by rationalizing it as an excuse to dress up, flaunt my assets, and allow myself to be fawned over by a member of the male persuasion, even when I knew their intentions were far from mine. It was a game no one really won; I'd dance, kiss, or exchange numbers with someone and allow it to go as far as I wanted, but by the next day the romance was gone and it was no longer as enticing.

Mating takes us back to our predatory roots. I've been the closest giraffe to a pack of carnivores, and much like in the wild, being in numbers doesn't always protect you. I was once dancing at a club with a group of my girlfriends when I felt something attach to my behind like a barnacle; a male, who decided the risk was worth taking, pounced on my ass and held on for dear life like a rodeo cowboy. Facing the opposite direction, my guard was down, and being several feet apart from this hormonally-driven male within a group of my own kind was not enough to deter him (I suppose my gyrating romp made him an offer he couldn't refuse). Luckily for me, my twentieth century defensive tactics were enough to confuse some sense of morality back into the leper; I stopped dancing, turned around to face him, and politely said

"I have a boyfriend."

I didn't, but the thought of conflict with another male was the appropriate tactic to appeal to this creature.

Think of a pigeon courting as he bobs his head up and down, slowly pacing closer and closer to the females. Without the benefit of an alluring plume, such as on the male peacock, he must use his wit and sheer persistence. The outcome is 50-50: either he is rebuffed or he succeeds in breaking the membrane, which allows others of his kind to float over and join in while the shields are down. If this one had made the kill, others of his kind would come to feast. On this animal planet we are all prey, and even when we're just trying to find some joy in life, we have to keep our wits about us.

Before going to a friend's party at a club downtown one night, Jem and I smoked up late in the evening, and I had already been wearing my contact lenses for most of the day. My eyesight is shit at the best of times, sporting a prescription so deep in the negatives that most eyeglass retailers laugh when I go in to buy a new pair. When I wear my glasses, the lenses are so thick that it becomes a party game to have my friends put them on and try to walk in a straight line. Society's beauty standards say the ugly girls are the only ones that can have shitty vision, but you can become hot instantly if you ditch the four-eyes. Because I like to masquerade as an attractive female, I preferred wearing my contacts when I went out. The trouble is, dry eyes are a common effect of smoking weed, and with foreign objects in them, they become particularly sensitive. Although I could normally ignore the tiny lenses floating around in my field of vision, while high, I was more attuned to their every movement in my eyes as they darted back and forth from my child-like wonder at everything and anything.

At the club, I couldn't help but put eye drops in at what seemed like every fifteen minutes, and I guess it started to draw attention. It's something nearly every stoner fears, driven to paranoia, that everyone can notice your red, squinty eyes and know that you are under the influence.

"Stop putting your eye drops in, you look like you're high!" Jem said (always looking out for me).

"Ok first of all, you know damn well I am—and second—I can't help it! My contacts are pissing me off!" I hissed. I was ready to claw my eyes out.

After the blessed drops of moisture had freshly bathed my eyeballs once again, the timer reset and fifteen minutes later I felt like I was looking through sand. This time I excused myself to the bathroom.

At the sink I clutched desperately to my small bottle of Aqua Vitalis and dropped one soothing tear at a time into my eyes. With the fire in one of my eyes out, I became aware of a shadowy presence at the entrance to the girl's bathroom.

"Are you high?" a man's voice called out from less than two feet away, the threshold between hallway and my safe haven thankfully respected.

What the fuck?! Did this guy follow me to the bathroom?

He was a lion, stalking me as I strayed from the herd.

I thought quickly despite the fear that triggered my survival instincts, and trying to sound un-intimidated, I casually released a drop into my other eye, as if barely registering the figure by the door before I replied.

"No, I've been wearing my contacts all day and they are *so* dry."

I sensed the man thinking about my answer as he stood there for another couple of seconds, and soon he disappeared as quickly as he came. I'm not sure what it was he was looking for: maybe he thought he could score some weed off of me, or maybe he was the stuff of warnings to young girls to be careful of men who prey on their lowered inhibitions. Either way, I was pleased that I had put on a good show of sobriety, and was able to produce a logical excuse followed through by a convincing act. I knew I would fight like a warrior to the end, using the natural defences nature has provided me against predators, like the six-inch pumps I was wearing at the time. I could barely walk in them, but I'd be able to maim someone real good.

It's horrifying to think that we may not have evolved past the days when all it took was a potato sack and a couple of buddies to go to the next settlement over and nab an unsuspecting bride. For the most part though, it's safe to say we *have* come a long way from our hunter-gatherer ancestors. Searching for a mate these days isn't quite the same as impressing the opposite sex by showing you can lift a heavier rock than other prospects, and since our brains have changed, so has the game. At least it's easier to recognize the production in my mind's high.

One particular night, the curtain was drawn back in an event I like the call the Bro Code Backfire. For those unfamiliar with the "Bro Code," it's an idea derived from the fictional character Barney Stinson on the popular American TV Show *How I Met Your Mother*. In the show, Barney is a so-straight-its-not-funny womanizer, often involved in multiple dalliances to the point that he has developed a system of etiquette for other heterosexual males to navigate friendships with their "bros" and what it means to be a man. This code is generally homophobic and derogatory to women, warning against acting like a "slut," "bitching," or ever wearing pink—although any offence I may have taken from this is replaced by the joy of irony, as Neil Patrick-Harris (the actor who portrays Stinson) is openly gay. The very first rule of the Bro Code is "Bros before Hoes"—a hoe being any woman that is not one's wife or direct family.

It's common knowledge that men want sex, and clubs become hunting grounds when females are out scantily-dressed with their defences down. The poison of choice is alcohol, which is sanctioned—even encouraged—in a place like this, and that night I was infected by both liquid and smoke. As Jem and I stumbled to the bar, we ordered drinks and were surrounded by a pair of wolves: one stood separate but remained close as his companion began to talk to me. We chat briefly in the superficial way one does with strangers, until there was a pause and I heard a voice behind me.

"Don't talk to that guy. He's an asshole."

I turned around to make eye contact with the owner of the voice, a dark-featured troll sitting nearby on a bar stool, looking at me with hooded eyes.

"How do you know he's an asshole?" I responded, taken aback by this random comment and wondering who the hell this guy was.

"Cuz I came here with him," he replied, "I know."

Either this guy was a terrible wingman or just very strange and awkward, but the intrusion raised my guard, and the audacity of telling me how to think put me on the defensive. If his icebreaker was to present his competition as inferior, he fumbled and the ball was caught by the other team.

The awkward silence was interrupted when Jem and I got our drinks, but we continued to talk with the "asshole" because he was cute. This made him far superior to his grumpy acquaintance, who offered nothing to the conversation after his brief interjection. Before long, the troll leaned over to whisper something to his asshole friend, and the two of them converged with a third (who materialized out of nowhere) to walk away without a backward glance or another word to either of us.

It seemed like I was a part in some sort of social experiment where the troll's attempt to deflect attention from his friend was supposed to entice curiosity toward himself. Perhaps the play was to present himself as superior and win the prize (namely Jem or I) but it backfired, and his wingman was inadvertently the winner. Replaying it in my mind, when he whispered in his bro's ear, I imagined the dialogue:

"Dude, that's not cool taking my kill like that. I like her, and it's easier for you to talk to women."

"Sorry bro, you're right—let's not fight. Neither of us will take her."

Or, it could have been as simple as:

"Yo—these bitches be crazy. Let's bounce."

Either way, it was bros before hoes. If only the animal kingdom were this cordial.

Although this event wasn't *entirely* fabricated by my mind, I am quite aware that the interpretation of the night's events could have been. It could have been Mad-Libbed, with all the silence as "fill in the blanks" to my inflated sense of hubris. Player B could have been the disgruntled brother of Player A who was buying all the drinks for the boys that night, and where the king goes the court follows. Or, I could have superimposed a poor plot line of a romantic Hallmark movie on to my experience. Alas, we'll never know–this is the brain on drugs after all– and sometimes the most trivial experience can seem like it's the scheme of something bigger. It's our mind's nature to make connections with new stimuli in an effort to compare it with our current knowledge, and then make connections to process it. It wouldn't be the first time the line between fantasy and reality would have merged in my adventures.

Under the influence of a high, if the smallest nuances of ordinary folk bore a striking similarity to those of celebrities, it didn't take long for my imagination to run wild. At a bar, a tall man with dark, curly hair cascading past his neck became Kit Harrington as his character Jon Snow (bastard son of Ned Stark and He-Who-Knows-Nothing), as it spilled over the collar of his burly winter cloak. The exaggerated features of Jim Carrey's countenance played on a stranger's face from the corner of a room, while I sauntered off to the dance floor with a ginger-haired man who became a shorter, less charismatic version of Tom Hiddleston. Jason Statham brushed past me, illustrated only by a square jaw, and a beard so faint that it appeared air-brushed. This was after I become convinced that I was talking with the singer Macklemore, whose identity was verified only by an identical hairstyle and a similar ethnicity. My mind ran with a mere pinch of suggestion during the times when Jem and I stumbled through the city fully in our intoxication, and it was all a heady mix of imagination, obsession, and desperation.

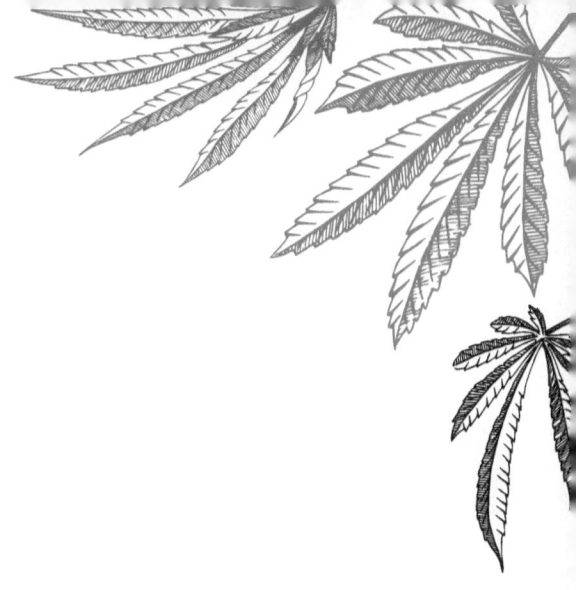

PART VII:
TO THINE
OWN SELF

30
Love And Obsession

When Jem broke up with Mike, her boyfriend of seven years, we had a more sombre Balcony Broads session, and I did the best I could to be there in her time of personal heartache. Desperate as I've been for a romantic partner, I've always clung hard to my independence, so although I had a few deep, platonic connections, I'd had even fewer romantic ones, which made it hard to relate to the depth of loss that Jem felt. I had always viewed men as a means to an end. For as long as I can remember, there's been a prehistoric part of my brain that remains focused on coupling, despite my inclination to choose being alone. This obsessive part of my genetic code was like a giant lizard—a crocodile whose eyes were always on the lookout for prey, ready to latch on and barrel roll an obsession to its demise. It existed for the singularly driven purpose of finding a romantic partner and dismissing the ones that don't appeal.

It was easy to develop insta-crushes and get carried away in daydreams when a high took hold, and I fondly ogled whatever creature stumbled into my view. Whenever Jem had one of her various male friends over, I would silently scrutinize them as the gears turned in my brain like an Asian matchmaker. On one occasion, neither of us listened to what they were saying, fixated as we were on their beautiful hair. Like a male version of the goddess Venus, it was impossible to tear our eyes away from the movement of his luxurious strands—neither too thick nor too thin—which were the colour of black obsidian, and bounced in perfect cadence to our conversation. It reminded me of celebrity Jared Leto and the fluidity of gender: despite being male, he would be equally as attractive as a female.

Trying to fit someone into the specific role of "The One" is a lot of pressure to put on a stranger—just think of how Neo initially refused to believe Lawrence Fishbourne's character in *The Matrix*. As a practicing Bud-dist, I tried to deconstruct the cause of my disappointments back to myself: approaching relationships with an expectation made it no one's fault but my own when they didn't live up to my ideals. This drew me further into myself to question my singular focus on the search for a soulmate.

The notion of a soulmate is a curious thing with many preconceived notions. The term is singular, implying everybody gets one in a lifetime, but if the soul is eternal, it crosses many lifetimes. Do we then assume to have the same mate each time, searching for them as they take different forms throughout different lives? Or do we open the assumption to multiple mates, straying from the notion that they are only romantic in nature? The former fit easily with my stubborn, close-minded sense of pride, but these days I'm more inclined to believe the latter. Sure, it may sound romantic, but when I started to critically analyze how the odds of finding that "one" out of a gazillion people across the world is nigh impossible, it seemed too cruel to be true. It makes more sense that we would have multiple matches across time and throughout our lives, and it would explain that odd feeling we sometimes get when we meet people and know subconsciously how we will get along even before we truly get to know them.

A mate is a match, and just as everyone has a "type" when it comes to romantic or sexual inclinations, there are friendships that last over others, and people in our lives that we feel more comfortable confiding in. These are the people we tend to keep around because they are easy to get along with and offer something meaningful and precious to our lives. By moving forward from the rigid belief of a soulmate only as a romantic partner, we untangle the neural wirings of our established beliefs and become free from limiting ideals. This allows the possibility of new relationships. In my case, it was a way to avoid disappointment by unfairly casting each wandering male as "potential husband number one" without a script.

While trying to convince myself a monogamous relationship was not on my mind, I had an opportunity to become sexually active with a guy who I knew had a girlfriend and wanted a discreet "friends with benefits" scenario. He was in business and seemed intelligent. Initially I was opposed, but ultimately unsure about my morality, as I was trying new things and trying to become more sexually aware. We would swap photos, and I rationalized to myself that it was just like porn; since guys in relationships watch porn (yes ladies, don't be fooled), it was no harm no foul.

There's no shame in trying something new in the search for happiness. After all, if you knew what made you happy, wouldn't you already be doing it? Until you find it, it makes perfect sense to change directions, and there is no wrong way. When you don't know where to start, the important thing is to trust that you'll learn along the way; take time with what serves you, and leave what doesn't. When you try to grow, you get to choose what direction to go in and you get to choose who you want to be.

Even though he kept trying to convince me that what his girlfriend didn't know wouldn't hurt her, my head and heart decided unanimously that I didn't want to play an active role in allowing someone to hurt another. I knew intimacy required a real commitment (as the Fresh Prince of Bel-air once taught me long ago), and sex seemed trivial in comparison to the importance of human compassion. How could compassion for others *not* be my concern? It was important to listen to my gut feeling and follow my truth, so I chose to concern myself with it, just as he chose to be unfaithful and untruthful to his partner. Why should my pleasure be built on someone else's betrayal? Why would

I want to propagate that sort of disrespect and keep that hurt alive? I declined his offer and chose to respect others, but more importantly, I chose to honour myself.

I continued to try and honour myself while remaining open to new experiences, but I found it extremely uncomfortable. Despite the desire I had for commitment, I always seemed to settle for the superficial and fleeting. I had a very eye-opening experience with a guy who was basically a "sex friend," and let me tell you, it's a very peculiar thing to meet a stranger twice: once when you are sober and once when you are under the influence of weed.

I had been seeing this guy who I wasn't particularly interested in, but he distracted me admirably. On one particular night I had invited him back to my place to see a movie with perfectly innocent intentions (how can you get to know someone if you never offer the opportunity after all?), and I played the perfect hostess to my guest:

"Can I offer you something to drink? A snack? A joint?"

This seemed to really excite him, and accepting the joint, we both indulged. Soon, his excitement level rocketed to a level of adolescence that I found off-putting.

"Is there more?" he asked me.

"Do you need more?" I answered back.

"I always need more, baby."

Ew.

Like alcohol, weed can lower any carefully crafted persona and reveal the kind of person that truly lies underneath. Heightened senses make it easier to detect red flags, and in that moment he not only became completely transparent to me, but also undesirable.

He had a flat face, lazy eyes, and a voice that was too high. He inflected words in ways that bothered me and used adolescent language like "chilling" with his friends, despite being well into his thirties. I realized he was very negative, and would needlessly comment on people we walked by. He was boring: always with the *Yakkaty Yak Yak* in a way that seemed stupidly ignorant. He also talked during movies.

After we smoked and decided on a movie to watch, he laid down on the couch and put his head in my lap; even though we had slept together numerous times, I was uncomfortable with the intimacy of it. Not only was there no longer any attraction, now there was fear. Fear of his touch and fear of his response to my rejection. I imagined asking him to leave. Even if he did leave, I was paranoid that he now knew where I lived, and that he might harass me with that information. I felt the fear of being afraid in my own home.

Through the reflection in the screen, I could see his eyes flutter and start to close, and I poked him to interrupt his slumber.

"What? I'm awake! I feel like I'm pissing you off."

Ah, there's the empathy kicking in, replaced quickly by anger. He stood up and suddenly got ready to leave.

Relief! Oh sweet justice he is leaving—and peacefully!

Carefully, I said nothing in protest, coming to the realization that I wanted him to go. It was unspoken and final, with no loose ends. I decided it was best to implement a new rule for myself: never get high on your own with a stranger; you need to feel safe or at the very least, have an easy exit.

Now blissfully alone, I relaxed in the glow of a fading sun above the city, while my thoughts wandered back to that inevitable, uncomfortable vortex of loneliness; the black hole that was my love life, ever present despite any number of available male celebrity obsessions I threw in. After the events of the day, I ruminated on my past failed relationships, and found an impartial, objective vantage point. Toke after toke, the situations shifted from shades of grey to a binary of black and white. I thought about all the warning signs and when I should have first noticed them, then broke the situations down objectively to cause and effect: X happened, so Y occurred. It's a strange feeling, analyzing your actions as an impartial judge, picking yourself apart and applying the past to the present with the investment of solving a tricky math problem. It brought me to a conclusion that I was thankful that these relationships were over.

Months later, my current *saveur du mois* was a real live boy (the most frustrating type), and this guy was as confusing as a damn calculus question. I had met him through a mutual friend, and goddamn he was beautiful. The past summer we had a date, which I thought went considerably well, but regrettably, the guy was a flake and our cordial conversations soon fell away. I moved on to the shady businessman I rejected, and the man-child who fell asleep during movies. As fate would have it, we met again much later at said mutual friend's birthday gathering and before you know it one thing led to another . . . I don't usually consider myself an aggressive person, but my crocodile companion was always prowling beneath the surface of my psyche, and they *are* predatory species.

I hadn't started using cannabis when I first met this man, and because I had by the time our paths crossed again, I was open to the strange working of the universe. It seemed like some twist of fate that we should have another chance together, so, misled by too many *Cosmo* magazines, I renewed my efforts for communication, thinking guys liked it when a woman was assertive.

Don't believe everything you read.

I managed to squeeze one more date out of the guy after our drunken hook-up: a pathetic dinner with one-sided conversation and discussion over some stupid Netflix TV show before we each paid our own bill and went our separate ways. I'm not bitter, I just thought it was supposed to go differently.

Crushing on a non-celebrity wasn't my usual modus operandi (although it did happen occasionally), and I found it was an especially awful thing to do when I was high. In my state of desperation, it was easy to grasp at straws that weren't there; it's hubris that swore when so-and-so smiled at me, they were really flirting. With my psychedelic imagination, pitting my crushes and I as star-crossed lovers was a dangerous game to play, and I hoped so much for something beyond my control that it was enough to break my own heart. Obsession can be compulsive, so it took a while for me to give up, but before I could let go, I had to realize when there was no possibility for something more from the relationship. I had to understand when I was wasting my time, and respect myself enough to know that I deserved better. Moving forward, I knew a positive relationship should be about compromise and balance, and whatever it was that I had with Mr. Calculus was clearly unbalanced. I didn't want to read into things anymore, and I was prepared for the truth, whether it was painful or not. I decided to put all my cards on the table.

I sent him a message on a popular social media platform (no one uses their phone to call anyone these days, it's too intimate), ready to get this shit over with. Despite my carefully constructed argument, it was like the high school equivalent of sending a note during class:

Do you like me? (Check 'Yes' or 'No')

Although I was notified the message was seen, he didn't respond.
Good riddance.
And then I met Carson.

31
Carson

With a lifetime of shyness as my default setting, the contradiction in personality was uncomfortable when my desire for a mate made me shameless and bold, and the repercussions weren't always felt until later when I reflected in embarrassment. Online dating seemed like a perfect fit for me because, like my celebrity crushes, I could investigate someone in my comfortable invisibility with the power of a search engine at the tips of my fingers. It's scary how easily personal information can be accessed with a little ingenuity and access to the internet, but this is how I met Carson.

They say a picture can tell a thousand words, and I was sold with a caveman's intrigue at a photo of his biceps, exposed like two shotgun barrels, as he delicately knelt down to do some gardening outside. Carson told me later about the planning that went into the picture when he told me about his three sisters, and how he enlisted their help for his photo shoot so he could have something to put on various dating profiles. He and I chatted back and forth for about a week, playing twenty-one questions, exchanging phone numbers, and texting each other when we weren't online. Even though I had been playing the online dating game for years, regardless of how desperate I was for a match, I always got anxious when things were moving well enough to consider meeting in person. It's easy to hide behind a persona from a screen and much more difficult to hide the truth of reality.

When we had talked long enough to get a sense of each other, I decided he intrigued me enough to agree to a date. During an exchange, I casually mentioned that I wasn't working, and that all I had planned for the day was a haircut. Within the hour my phone rang showing an unknown number.

My gut knew what was happening before my brain caught up–I wasn't used to the boldness of male pursuit. I answered my cell phone.

"Hello?"

"Hey! It's Carson," a deep, excited voice said on the other end.

"Oh! Hey?"

"Do you know when you'll be finished with your appointment? I'm on my way downtown now and should be there in twenty minutes."

I didn't know what to say, torn between shock and fear.

First of all, who calls anyone anymore??
Second, holy assumption, Batman.
And third, do you know how long women's haircuts take?!

I told him it would take at least an hour and that I hadn't even left my apartment to go to the salon yet. Despite my swirling anxiety, I was interested in him, so I decided to overlook the potential stalker behaviour and see its flattering side: how he was so excited to meet me that he dropped everything to rush over, vying for a piece of my time. He would have to wait for me, but he seemed eager, and you know what they say about good things that come with patience. It's also true what they say about those special relationships: you'll know when you find them.

Our first date was like something out of a movie. I left the hair salon with a pep in my step (in no small part due to my fancy 'do), and finding his number in my recently-called list, I dialed, anxious by our upgrade from text-to-voice in such a fast period of time. I told him I was finished, and where to meet me. Since my female survival instincts were on point, I picked a busy street to meet for the safety in the open. Soon enough, he was running across the street dressed in a leather jacket overtop a "Bazinga" shirt (it was his attempt to look cool while appealing to my inner nerd that I'd talked so much about). He looked especially nervous in front of me, but surprisingly, I felt calm. Unfortunately, the guns were holstered due to the cold weather; I would have liked to meet them too.

We went for coffee in a cozy cafe a few steps away from our meeting point, and chatted as the sun shone through the windows of the cafe to light up our eyes. The conversation was easy, and we quickly became comfortable with each other long after our coffee cups sat empty and forgotten. During the easy silence, I vouched in blunt honesty:

"This is going pretty well, huh?!"

Momentarily left speechless (a rarity, I would discover later), he smiled.

Once the sun began to set, we left the cafe and ventured down the street, stopping into a gem store that I mentioned I liked to go to once and a while. It was really an excuse to prolong each other's company. He dominated the conversation, and over-shared everything—like how he once got hit in the balls so hard during hockey that he peed blood for a couple days. He had inadvertently put his own life in danger in a pool mishap. He was sexually molested as a child. Simultaneously angry at himself for his verbal diarrhea but unable to stop talking, he thought he blew his chance for a second date early on, but as a quiet person who talked very little, I was grateful for him to carry the conversation. I was also highly entertained.

As we looked around the gem store he pointed to a small bowl of wish stones, each inscribed with a single word, and asked me which I liked the most. I sensed an ulterior motive to his question but humoured him, pointing to a blue goldstone (a crystal said to help wisdom, energy, and courage) with the word "hope" on it. Hope was something that had played a large part in my life and past relationships. We circled the store for a bit longer, and then left.

Unfamiliar with the downtown streets, Carson forgot where he parked his car. It was a cold night in early winter, and I walked with him to navigate the tightly packed suburban neighbourhood in the settling darkness. Finding the familiar street, we walked past a cat standing on a porch with its paws on the door of a house as if trying to look in. It looked over its shoulder as we approached, and meowed before coming over to weave itself, shivering, in between our legs. We knocked on the door of the house, thinking that it lived there and was trying to get in, but the lights were off, and it seemed no one was home. I picked the little guy up and put him inside my coat to keep him warm: he was small, but looked older than a kitten, and the name on his collar said "Felix." I supposed his curiosity in the outdoors got the best of him this night, and he was quickly regretting it.

Carson called the phone number we found on his collar. At first there was no answer, but driven by the cold and the kitty's wellbeing, we called until someone eventually picked up. It turned out Felix didn't even live at the house where we found him, but at one down the street. Running to get his car, Carson pulled it up beside me, and with the cat warmly stowed against my breast, we drove several feet down the street to the house Felix did belong to. We handed him off to a stout, mildly embarrassed man who smiled and explained how this was not the first time the cat had wandered off—for some reason he tended to get his houses confused.

After the rescue, Carson and I sat in the warmth of the car with the adrenaline aftermath. Our egos were bloated, and we felt good about ourselves now that our good deed of the day was done. We were also hungry after the excitement, so our date turned from a mild-mannered meet-and-greet with coffee, into dinner.

It was later now, and the sun had sunk deeper against the sky making the night even colder, so we drove to the closest main street and parked parallel to the sushi restaurant we chose. After opening the passenger side door for me, I ogled as he removed his glasses to put them in a case inside the door's side compartment. His eyes were a pale blue, intense against the contrast of his red shirt. He kind of looked like a stumpier version of Nathan Fillion, and gained +20 in sexy.

Even though the conversation in the restaurant remained mostly one-sided on his end, I was lapping it up. I always preferred listening to talking. I took a quick visit to the bathroom before the bills arrived, and when I returned he had already paid, and the mood had shifted: He was silent, with eyes downcast and a serious look on his face. Speaking slowly, he said he was having a wonderful time, and then reached into his pocket.

"I *hope* we can have a second date," he said, coyly placing the shimmering blue stone I had picked out earlier at the gem shop on top of the table. The word hope, in proud gold letters, stared up at me.

Well played, sir. Well played.

As I was grinning from ear to ear like an idiot, Carson described his unspoken mission with the store clerk to buy the stone, and I envisioned the silent transaction as it was explained to me: picking up the stone without me noticing, he circled the store repetitiously to establish eye contact with the cashier and nodded to him, pointing a finger to my back as I looked around obliviously. Without hesitation, the cashier met his nod with one of his own, and on Carson's next circle back to the counter, the cash was flashed and exchanged without a word. I silently thanked the store clerk in my mind, feeling that he was the true hero of the day.

After dinner, Carson drove me down the street the short distance to my apartment, and we both got out of the car to say goodnight. Approaching the door to the lobby, he held it open for me.

"I had a great time tonight," he said. "I'm not going to kiss you, but I hope we can get together again soon . . ."

Unacceptable.

"Well, *I* am" I said, and grabbed him by the shirt collar to plant a big wet one on his lips, which were unresponsive due to the apparent shock.

I pulled away, smiling at his dumbfounded expression, and watched as he started to walk back toward his car in a daze. It's nice to have that effect on someone.

He stopped after a few paces and turned back to me, muttering to himself as much as me under his breath.

"Once more," he said, with his finger pointing up at me, even though his eyes were unfocused on the ground.

Coming out of his stupor, they snapped up to meet mine as he took my face with both hands and kissed me. It was a life-changing kiss—seriously—my knees went weak and everything.

The rest, as they say, was history.

32
Life With Carson

If there's one thing that is constant in life, it's change, and for better or worse, change is inevitable. Sometimes we try to ignore it, avoiding it with self-constructed blinders as we trot down paths laid before us, and other times we race towards it, eager for its unfamiliarity. Most of the time, we don't discover until after we've changed paths, how it has affected our lives. In quiet moments it's interesting to line up the dominoes and see how they fell to create the lives we live today.

Up until the Carson Era, Jem and I felt our lives had been going opposite to how we expected. Just like when we used to play with Barbies as kids, we always thought I would be the one that would settle down in a relationship while she remained single and exploratory. Thus far, my adventures with cannabis had focused my goals toward self-discovery and reflection, while she remained with Mike. In some cosmic twist, with our souls entwined as they were, Jem broke up with Mike on the very day I met Carson.

Carson and I moved quickly, infatuated with one another and the singular focus we both had on starting a life together. We met in January so our first Valentine's Day was still early on in our relationship, and we went hard and fast. He picked me up at my apartment, dressed in the new outfit he helped pick out and pay for, and brought me to a summer house that his parents owned. Even though the days were turning brighter, we were still in the middle of our Canadian winter and the ice refused to leave easily, clinging to the pavement as he led me, blindfolded, from the warmth of his car to the warmth of rustic wood.

Inside, he removed the silk covering my eyes and gestured to a small coffee table in the corner of the room. The glass tabletop had a set of bowls, plates, and cutlery. A bottle of wine sat on its glossy surface.

"You'll be having dinner here, madam" he said in his best English butler voice.

I was led to the table, and sat down while he shuffled into the adjacent room. He returned with a bowl of soup, a red creamy colour, and set it down in front of me before disappearing once again into the back. I dipped my spoon shallowly into the liquid, taking an edge and bringing it to my mouth. It was cold, and it tasted like tomato.

He made me cold tomato soup.

I shrugged internally. (They say it's the thought that counts?)

He surprised me after dinner with chocolates, and a candle-lit bath at the end of a path covered in rose petals; I supposed his love language was 'acts of service'. Growing up, whenever I visited my dad, he would buy me the things that I wanted as a way to show he cared, so naturally, my love language manifested as 'gift-giving'. My gift to Carson was a heart made out of rose quartz (to mirror the crystal he gave me on our first date), and I decorated the wooden box I put it in with lyrics from the love songs that reminded us of one another. I wrote a letter in my usual expressive manner, explaining how I had been waiting my whole life for him (blah blah blah), and how he had my heart (get it?) until the day I died.

I was welcomed easily by his family, his three sisters and his mom and dad who, unlike mine, were still married. Despite their acceptance, my inclusion was strange and uneasy because it was so different from what I was used to. Family dinners, family game nights, and talking about each other's days were foreign to me. I was happy to be a part of it, but I felt like an imposter. It would take years for me to learn to open up to them, let alone to feel that I was deserving of the acceptance they so freely offered.

To herald the start of spring, our unofficial national animals–the cobra chicken–migrated back to us, as the trees and grass blushed green into life. People were outdoors more, and Jem and I could finally go out on our porch without jackets. It was Kitkat that first noticed the change, flirting with me whenever Carson wasn't around, as if she sensed the shift in my priorities and attempted to right them. I was overjoyed by my new relationship and declared triumphantly to friends that I'd found "Him"— that elusive One that I'd been hunting for as long as I could remember. I knew a new chapter of my life was opening, and I was eager to dive in.

After travelling for the first time together, Carson and I decided to move in with one another five months after we met. Despite the several years Jem and I had lived together re-discovering our childhood friendship, I was infatuated with my new romance and over the span of a couple months, Jem and I went our different ways. Now that she had uncoupled from Mike, she moved to the United States where she spent her summers as a child, to start anew. I moved on to a new nursing job, and remained blissfully distracted from my frustration with the profession by my new relationship. I also started to drive, and although I had grown accustomed to the city as a pedestrian, the city soon lost its appeal to me, and was replaced by impracticality and frustration.

I found my once familiar life behind me, swept up by the ultimate focus of my love life and the notion that I had shifted from one soulmate to another. Now that I was away from the haven Jem and I once reigned over in the sky, the world looked different. I was no longer out on top of the world with my sister-in-spirit, bundled up against the world above the lights and sounds of the inner city below us. The apartment Carson and I rented had a balcony, but now I snuck outside on my own to smoke, and was surrounded by identical outcrops that stuck out like the teeth of a colony ship from some science fiction movie. My new neighbours and I were uncomfortably close, and I felt like we had become caged animals in a zoo, separated by concrete and chicken wire. We were all guarded chihuahuas trying to face our lives bravely:

all sound and fury as we tried to carve out our lives in this vast universe. As time passed, the honeymoon phase of my relationship faded, and even though I thought I found the man of my dreams, I started to feel more alone than ever.

Carson had the personality of a popular, retired Hollywood actor that's finding it hard to give up the spotlight: self-assured in his world views, and hesitant to change with the times. He could be incredibly stubborn to the point where it came across as pretentious. Despite peer pressure, he had never gotten high or felt the need to discover what cannabis might have to offer him. Although I respected his opinion to abstain, as well as his general acceptance of my use, it was hard not to feel judged by him.

Even though we were past the days of trying to hide any unbecoming habits from each other in fear of rejection, I found myself trying to hide when I got high because I could feel his discomfort (real or imagined) like a cloud over me. Over time, he became more accepting of the importance of weed in my life, but it was still hard not to bring my high out into the open. I liked it better when he couldn't tell. Thankfully, being the truest version of myself with him, he often never knew I was under the influence unless I mentioned it.

It was an uncomfortable feeling to hide such a sensitive part of who and what I was: a spiritual seeker, learning to embrace imperfections as proof of my individuality. I was offended by Carson's inability to see weed as anything but the tool I saw it as, because I mirrored his fervour. Part of the reason getting high with Jem was so healing was because we had grown up together, and had a history so deep and rich in experiences, that we didn't judge each other.

I snuck outside to smoke in the shadows, on the foreign balcony of the first apartment Carson and I lived in together. After weeks of being sober, I was eager to regain the part of myself I was missing. When I felt myself rising upwards into the comforting arms of my higher self, it was like greeting an old friend:

"Sup, Brah! Where have you been??"
"I've been in love down on Earth, dude."
"Oooooo, righteous!"

It was a positive affirmation in the times of uncertainty.

Carson would find me sometimes on the balcony, gently swaying side to side, and I felt immediately vulnerable, as if caught by my parents doing something I wasn't supposed to.

"Are you hiiiiigggh?" he said, poking me gently in the shoulder like a child with a stick, unsure of how to approach a new creature.

"I'm about an 8 ½ to a 9 out of 10" I replied, thinking to myself as I looked at him:

Dude. You need a haircut.

High or sober, I always felt my advice went unheeded.

Considering the similarities between Carson and I, and the effect cannabis had on me, I wished he would have tried it. I respected his choice not to, of course, but my experience as a Balcony Broad made me eager to connect in his company the same way. He and I were cut from the same cloth, and I felt that it would help him discover a direction in life—perhaps even a purpose—which was something I knew we both craved. My trips led me to greater expression and a need to write, which pulled out the silent child that grew up under her own thumb. I figured with some psychedelic insight, he could learn to get out of his own way too. That being said, with his love of food and eating, even though I wished he could re-discover the lust for food when high, I was afraid that he might literally eat himself to death.

I regressed, faced with the emotional discomfort from the absence of Jem and the harsh reality that Carson couldn't fill the space that she did. Smoking weed was no longer a recreational activity, or a bonding experience with another soul, and despite my desire to hold on to the habit because of the insight it provided, my highs became unpredictable rollercoaster rides. Anxious and worried about the future, I wasn't prepared for the emotions I faced without someone who knew what I was going through to talk me down. High or sober, I felt that as a male, there were things my mate could not simply relate to when faced with the clusterfuck of the female brain, hormones, and the psychoactive effects of cannabis that shakes them together with the unpredictability of a Magic 8-ball. I didn't feel safe or indestructible anymore. The rose-coloured lenses were gone, darkened by the stress of the physical world.

Developing health issues slowly during the years Carson and I lived together, Kitkat got sick. I was sitting on my bed, wasting time on my phone before I had to go into work for an evening shift, when I heard her uneasy chirrup from behind the bedroom door. I got up and opened it to see her sitting outside, and my heart dropped when I saw how much effort it required for her to get from sitting to standing to enter the room. I immediately scooped her up, and Carson and I drove straight to the emergency vet clinic in town. Her issues had come to a head, insidiously planting cancer in her bowels to the point there was no treatment available to keep it at bay anymore. Now, it was time to say goodbye–I wouldn't let her suffer. I was there until the bitter end, taking solace in the belief that she knew even when her eyes closed for the last time, I would still be there.

Parts of my old life continued to fall away, while little good took its place. My role as a nurse continued to weigh me down, my soul sisters were gone, and despite having a good man, I continued to feel alone. And yet, I felt desperate to stay in a relationship. I knew I wanted to get married one day, but I was hesitant to commit myself to Carson, considering how I was starting to feel unfulfilled by what we had. Like a typical man, he wasn't sure about marriage either, and would often voice his concern over the need to seal a relationship like a contractual obligation. While this used to bother me before when I craved commitment, I grew complacent with his view and never fixated on whether he would ever propose or not—I had a lot to work through.

Remember when I mentioned one of my love languages was gifts? Both of my parents indulged Adam and I in this way, and even though both of our birthdays were close to Christmas, we always got gifts for each occasion. When Carson and I started dating, he rarely marked special occasions with gifts, saying that he didn't believe it was a way one should show love. It bugged me initially, but eventually I let it go to respect his difference of opinion. For my mom, it was a different story, and she would *harrumph* in displeasure whenever she asked what he got me for my birthday, and I had to admit it was nothing except a warm acknowledgement.

For this reason, I should have known that something was up when Carson planned a trip to Aruba—all expenses paid by him, despite my desire to help—and said it was my birthday and Christmas present in one. He was clever to rely on the timing for it to seem innocent; he wanted it to look like a coincidence, instead of the bright flag it usually signals for spontaneous proposals. Going so far as to plan the trip around a full moon (so it would be bright when he took me for a walk on the beach), I was completely oblivious, only cluing in when we stopped on our walk, and his hand went to his pocket.

"I love you," he said simply, opening the small jewellery box he pulled out containing my engagement ring. "I want to spend the rest of my life with you."

I was surprised by the disappointment I felt when he didn't get down on his knee like I had seen in every romantic drama of my life. He explained later that it was because bowing to someone seemed like an act of surrender to him, and God forbid he give up control of any kind.

I said yes, and at the time it happened, I was ready to put aside the imperfections of our relationship and start down the path society lays for all women: to get married, have kids, and suppress any further desire for self-discovery by deflecting my needs in favour of the care of others. For the six years Carson and I were together, I was slowly drawn to this moment—faced with what I thought I always wanted—and I was oblivious to the anchor it hooked onto my feet. Sometimes sad truths are only apparent after we get what we think we wanted.

33
Moving On

Then came an unimaginable change in the tide, and a worldwide pandemic forced Carson and I closer together than we had ever cared to be. For six years, the part of myself that practiced quiet remained a dominant part of my personality, and I was fine deferring to him as my "other half." How could he be wrong since he was who I'd been looking for my entire life? I was finally in a relationship that lasted, and most of the time, our views brought us to agree on the same actions. For the most part I was always able to retreat with myself, recharging like a typical introvert, but now, forced inside during a quarantine with nowhere to go, I felt suffocated. I needed room to breathe, but every time I turned around, he was there, distracting me from the desire to find myself.

Life accelerated during the pandemic—in no small part due to the insurmountable stress that continued in my nursing profession—and the person I was carefully incubating in isolation started to spill over. Even though I wasn't living with Jem anymore, indulging in cannabis was something I didn't give up; how could I when it helped me so much? I *liked* who I was in the haze of the high, and my confidence grew in my spirituality. Meanwhile, Carson's mind remained closed to it all, dismissing it casually as "woo woo." Our minds didn't seem to work the same way anymore, and even though I was the kind of person to give benefit of the doubt, he remained stubborn. I had moved past the earlier version of myself, fixed in her ways and snide toward anything that didn't fit with her view of the world, but he didn't, and continued to judge others with differing beliefs as inferior. I was still living with the past, but thankfully, I realized I was growing forward.

As I did my personal, introspective work and learned to face the parts of myself that held me back, I started to resent the way he acted with the booming sound of thunder, and the soft flash of lightning. To me, all I saw was talk, and no follow-through. A self-saboteur. A hypocrite out of ignorance. But worst of all, he made me feel stupid. He made me doubt myself, convinced that his way was the only way that made sense. I started to disentangle myself from him, but it was with the ease of Velcro.

I became hardened to the nuances of the person I fell in love with. Without the rose-coloured glasses of infatuation, although the love never left, reality rolled in like clouds on a sunny day foreboding rain. It was the small things that triggered me the most, despite how frivolous they seemed, because it trivialized how deeply I was affected. When he moved my things without asking, he often forgot where he put them, and when I confronted him about it, he said it made better sense for them to be where he decided. My opinion didn't seem to matter. Although I was happy with this arrangement at the beginning of our relationship (I was the messy one, determined that cleaning was often an exercise in futility), it slowly became to feel like blatant disrespect. My individuality suffered.

When the honeymoon phase had run its course, Carson and I seemed to devolve in to that of Ashton Kutcher and Brittany Murphy's relationship in *Just Married,* a movie that breaks the Disney stereotype of Happily Ever After by representing the other 60-70% of couples in the world. Proving the old adage about common sense not being so common, it captures the discomfort of realizing what it truly means to be intimate with someone, and how romance gets interrupted by the uncomfortable truth that relationships take work.

This was especially difficult to confront when all my life I'd felt that a special someone would help me put all the pieces of an elusive happiness together: a scapegoat to hoist all my future dreams and happiness upon. After the dust settled and the infatuation disappeared, I had trouble coming to terms with reality. Despite our moral similarities, I couldn't help but feel a sense of loss over the fact that I'd never be able to develop as intense a relationship with Carson as I had with Jem, my best friend. Like some great cosmic joke, he faced me as an earlier version of myself, who was stubbornly prideful and cynical, bringing to life the saying "be careful what you wish for."

I continued to bite my tongue, chasing the promise of happiness through romantic partnership, but I was starting to grow out of that belief now that my retreat into independence was making a comeback. I realized there is no "One" that could fix everything that makes me uncomfortable in life. Carson certainly couldn't do it, no matter how many tries I gave him, or the amount of excuses I made to myself that it would get better since love was all we needed.

Whenever I met my higher self through smoking, it seemed like she could predict the future with a clairsentience that I never knew, and she saw that our time together was ending. It was like the universe was sending me signs: when I was reading tarot cards, meditating, or doing anything for myself and by myself, he would always invade. Whether it was the crack of light coming in from an open door or the shrill sound of my phone when he called me after he got off work every day, I felt interrupted. I felt like I could never be completely whole if he kept pushing his way in. At first I fought it, but like a child growing in the womb, the space in which to grow became too small, and it wasn't long before the uncomfortable pains of confinement became too much to be ignored.

What was lacking became more apparent as the months together drew on, and eventually I convinced myself that this was it—nothing was going to change. My time alone was freedom, and I wanted more of its nourishing touch, but I was afraid of what there was out there on my own. Six years of companionship is a hard thing to break no matter what. As much as I tried to hide it with him, he could notice the change in me. He could tell I was becoming distant, avoidant, and less engaging. Eventually I was able to open up and tell him how I was feeling, but I was further annoyed that the conversation brought me to tears while his eyes remained dry as bone. The same pattern repeated for months: him noticing the distance, me talking about how I felt, him striving to do better, striving and stopping, then the distance. Then, it was like one day I had simply woken up, and things had changed for me past the point of return.

When we still believed the pandemic would resolve in time for our wedding, we planned our engagement photos. It was odd to step backwards, into the role of being wholly in love after all that had passed. Our photographer was wonderful, and he made us both feel as ease, but my smiles didn't feel authentic, and I feared even worse: that they may have just been an act. As we stood on an outcrop of the beach we shot at, we were alone while our photographer took our pictures from afar. Carson looked at me in a way I could barely remember—his eyes were soft, and so full of love. As he touched my face tenderly, I saw how plain his feelings were, and the guilt sat in my stomach with the weight of a boulder.

My restless soul sought to get away, so I planned a trip to Algonquin Provincial Park (I informed Carson that I was going, and that it *would* be nice if he came too, but his decision wouldn't sway mine). It was a cleansing trip, and the location had a small meditation hut full of items that the land's owner, a shaman, had accumulated over years. I sat inside, feeling the sun as it warmed me through the windows, surrounded by relics of the earth, and totems made from the nature that surrounded us. Clay, softened from the moisture of the lakes, had been moulded to represent creatures that shared the land with us: snake, turtle, wolf, bear . . . those that symbolized the characteristics we desire in life: healing, transformation, wisdom, perseverance, freedom, courage. Being in nature teaches us to be still and to not feel guilty for it. Instead of trying to prove our worth to the world, we can reflect on what has stood to exist longer than we have, and will continue to stand long after we are gone.

The great irony of our ego is revealed in nature: although we may have the most evolved mammalian brains, our intellect can be an obstacle which keeps us from enjoying the simplicities of life that bring the most pleasure. Often, we look outwards to find a purpose while ignoring the acceptance that we can only find from within ourselves. Learning hard truths helps us grow the most.

Carson and I made it official on our trip, coming to an understanding that as a romantic relationship, there was no benefit for either of us. We were always good friends, and eventually became great roommates, but with a growing spirituality that he could not nurture, I grew up and away. It seemed like a blessing in disguise that we could drop the pretense and loosen our belts. I felt like I could breathe again.

34
Growing Forward

I've learned more about myself than I ever thought I could through the relationships I've had with those closest to me, and cannabis has made this possible. I'm learning to feel confident in my eccentricities, even though this inflated sense of confidence scares me and goes against everything I have been up until now. It's still hard, but I'm learning to believe in myself. If there's one thing video games have taught me in life, like in *The Sims* (a real-life personality simulation game) you can always start over. If your Sim tries to experiment in the kitchen with insufficient cooking skill points and ends up setting themselves on fire, you too, can load from the last save point and decide that maybe ordering pizza for dinner is a better decision until you're ready to try again. Practice makes perfect.

I accessed to my subconscious through my cannabis use in the way Carlin alluded to when he recognized the cognitive dissonance within himself. Like exercising a muscle, the more practice I had, the deeper I was able to go by stretching the most under-used parts of my brain. The psychedelic effect of cannabis drew me inward to acknowledge decades of suppressing of my wants, needs, and desires from childhood—whether I liked it or not. I created my own trauma as a child, justifying my independence as strength when all I wanted was to feel deserving of love. By being afraid of rejection, I retreated from others, and avoided opening up to my emotions.

Despite the paradox, I was a solitary creature looking for connection. I was so focused on trying to find "the One" that would understand me, that I never stopped to think that what I was really looking for was self-acceptance and the encouragement to know that I was good enough. I was waiting for my life to be completed by another person, but I understand now that it won't be. It simply *can't* be.

People are flawed by nature, and honestly, the sooner you realize that, the easier life becomes. It's similar to growing up and realizing that your parents are simply people; despite how omnipotent they seemed to you as a child, they were just making it up as they went along. And so are we as we come to understand that nobody is perfect, because there is no such thing as perfection.

Relationships aren't guaranteed a "happily ever after," because life doesn't end with a pretty little bow. You are still you—imperfections, trauma, and all—and despite any compliment someone can bring to you, any unhappiness will resurface if you've never faced it at its source. There's an old saying: to love someone, you must learn to love yourself first. The idea is simple, suggesting that before you can be free to experience genuine love for another being, you need to first find it within yourself. Explained by Osho, an Indian guru and leader of a controversial spiritualist movement that combines philosophy and religion:

"The capacity to be alone is the capacity to love. It may look paradoxical to you, but it's not. It is an existential truth: only people who are capable of being alone are capable of love, of sharing, of going into the deepest core of the other person—without possessing the other, without becoming dependent on the other, without reducing the other to a thing, and without becoming addicted to the other. They allow the other absolute freedom because they know that if the other person leaves, they will be as happy as they are now. Their happiness cannot be taken by the other person because it is not given by the other."

The means to this story's end (TLDR) is a proposal, and a challenge to the current rhetoric on drugs. Considering the current debates surrounding marijuana and it's legalization across the Western world, I propose a view that being high is not always about trying to escape reality, but more about trying to experience and embrace life as a verb rather than just a noun. In Bud-dism, still waters run deep.

A life of mediocrity nudged me toward spiritual escapism, and my intention was to ignore the traumas of my past, skipping right to the easy part of living a fulfilled life. Unfortunately, that's not the way our minds work. There are no short-cuts in life when you want a quality outcome. Personal growth depends on processing the muck of painful emotions to move past them.

One of the most important reasons behind this endeavour is to share what pushed me past my elitist mentality, and to offer a narrative on positive experiences with marijuana or cannabis, from someone who used to be vehemently against any recreational form of drug. When I opened myself up to change looking for a direction in life, I initially sought fungi ('shrooms) but explored foliage instead, and I wouldn't have allowed myself to experiment with either of these while in my old way of thinking. I digress that all searches for the truth need to have an element of risk to them, but I don't mean to imply that you must hit rock bottom before you can find your way back up. Although mushrooms DO grow in the dark, like plants, we need to be nurtured by the light.

Spirituality is embedded in the practice of science and evolution. As a species, we survived by adapting to our environment, and the more we learned, the more we evolved; when our ancestors created the wheel, it changed our world, and the growth of our minds ensured our continued survival. As the ability of our minds grew, we established modern psychology as we know it today: the learning about the learning of the mind. We seek to understand it, in the hopes that it may provide some vital clue to understanding ourselves, and our place in the universe.

Spirituality is also the love child of psychology and philosophy. As the mind perceives, perception creates experiences, and experiences produce life. Since we experience the world through the mind, this is just like the famous philosophical question: If a tree falls in a forest and no one is around to hear it, does it make a sound?

Can the world exist without a mind to perceive it? Can the mind exist if there is no world for it to exist in?

Pair that with the cornerstone of modern philosophy from René Descartes: I think, therefore I am. There can be no thinking without a mind to do it, and for this reason we can be assured of our existence. Our existence now conjures the self.

By studying our minds, we discover ourselves. How we perceived experiences in our minds laid the groundwork for our psyches, and the responses to these life experiences shaped our personality traits to create who we are. Imagine what we could then do with the power to rewrite our lives by becoming self-aware? By realizing this, our continued existence—and what that looks like—is up to us.

"To study the Buddha way is to study the self"
Dogen Zenzi (Old Buddhist guy)

In my own Bud-a'way, the psychedelic effects of cannabis broke down psychological barriers, opening me to spiritual consciousness, a sense of peace within myself, and a death of the ego. Whether it be a part of the plan of a divine being or some unexplainable coincidence, the blood of this earth offers us a spiritual tool: a chemical compound that allows us to turn inward and study ourselves, rather than put the onus on the outward physical world that we've evolved to judge.

We are no longer our barbaric ancestors. Our minds are more powerful, and we have developed the world around us into something we don't even recognize at times. Just as we have survived and grown exponentially, our needs have grown and changed, too. It's no longer enough to simply survive, we need purpose—but not in the way society would have us believe.

A purpose is not just a reason for living, it's a direction. What direction do you want to steer your life in? If the mind and the world are one, let's test a theory and try to exercise some level of control: What would your life look like if you knew which path led you to your greatest happiness? But how can you discover what will make you happy if you don't really know or understand yourself?

Whether we come from different parts of the world or different cultures, speak different languages or believe different things, we all (even the assholes of the world) want the same thing: to be happy. By delving into your own mind, you can face your so-called negative traits and appreciate the positive ones. Get to know what makes you tick and try to discover why. Get rid of the victim mentality and learn to recognise the patterns of bad scenarios so you can take different actions to avoid the same mistakes; pull your head away from the wall you're banging on to discover the window above you.

Like me, you could spend your whole life thinking things will always get better once you find him/her/it aka The One, and that your life will finally be complete. But just as I had to realize the unrealistic expectations I was thrusting upon strangers, we all have to discover that no one can help us achieve our dreams but ourselves—not from a lack of wanting to, but from the sheer impossibility of it.

Find yourself. Even if you exist in a relationship with another, plan a life outside of your partner's by enjoying the things that you do, and enjoy being yourself. I used cannabis as a tool to extend my reach inward, initially through journaling, but the trail of breadcrumbs I left myself while high always took me back to a place of mind where I was free to be loose and cool, self-confident and free. To express myself in any way came naturally through my writing and freed all thoughts from my mind.

Forget what society has taught you to be right (God forbid we talk about our feelings or the matters that are truly important to us, am I right?). We should stop putting so much goddamn pressure on ourselves and others, pull up our bootstraps, and heal from the inside out.

When we are able to access the root of our perceptions, we can analyze them, and as our minds expand, we can grow into better versions of ourselves. When we all grow as individuals, a funny thing happens where we stop focusing so much on ourselves (our flaws, the what-if's, and the jealous comparisons) and become interested in others. By dismantling your ego, you might find a higher purpose.

With the ego aside, we can discover common ground and become comfortable sharing ourselves with others. What inevitably follows is the ultimate knowledge that always hides in plain sight: we're all just trying to get through this life with minimal burn damage like Mario, the little-plumber-that-could, to find our version of the princess in the castle—a reason to go on. I bare my soul to urge you to explore humility, to learn to evolve from experiences—past and present— and to seek peace and fulfilment in your life. Judging brings you nothing, while learning opens the world to you. Learn about life, each other, and those around you instead of denying them of any value out of fear.

Ironically, there is great power in learning to be vulnerable with others, but because there's always a fear of rejection, it takes courage to get to that point. I'm still learning that I'm not as alone in the world as I feel: we are all the same, *and* we are all different. We simply exist as a presence to be felt by others. Find your truth, discover your wisdom, and appreciate life and each other.

In the end, I guess I did get a vision:

Spread-eagle, human beings are all shaped like stars.

Maybe if we all try to sparkle together, we can be as equally brilliant as the night sky.

Nothing like leaving on a high note.

Epilogue

It took me a decade to write this book, and it took even longer to share it with those outside my close circle and revise it to make any sort of sense to the general reader (but the jury is still out on that I suppose). From the generation of the first draft, to putting it down and picking it back up again, it took determination and a belief in myself that I didn't even know I possessed. For years, I struggled to put the work in to this project that needed to be done, but despite the lack of motivation, whenever I returned to it, the story grew and my voice got louder. Aside from that, it took the passage of time to realize that instead of blaming myself for its incompletion after all that time, it literally couldn't have been finished until enough time, and certain things, had come to pass.

I miss the reign of the Balcony Broads, and I'll never forget the treasured moments like the pissing contests between Jem and KitKat:

"Meow!"
Jem: "Don't you judge us!"
"Meow."
Jem: "That's right."
"Meow . . ."
Jem: "Oh no you *didn't*! Gurl, hold mah earrings . . ." (to me)

To truly be a memoir, there has to be a beginning and an ending, with the promise of an epilogue. I was still with Carson in my original ending, but now I know the completion of this book before now would have been impossible. Just like in nature, with death comes the birth of something new. A tree grows from a seed in the dirt using the resources surrounding it, and the sun and the rain nourish it. If the conditions are good it receives life—growing tall and bold—while it gives life in return to organisms like moss and fungi which attach to it and thrive. When the tree dies, it becomes fuel for the new life of flames, or its skeleton can remain, providing shelter to smaller creatures. If my romance with Carson was like a tree, it had died, but with the acceptance of its demise our friendship could blossom, as if the dying ends of our engagement were fed back into the circle of life. A new type of connection grew, and he remains one of my closest friends to this day.

It was truly a matter of divine timing: life laying out the dominoes until the time I decided enough was enough. My breakup was the catalyst I needed to push myself that last little bit of the journey, through barriers that were physical, vibrational, or otherwise, to realize that I am my One, and I have everything I need to grow strong.

Like recording a piece of advice for later remembrance, this note-to-self is my experience to share with you, with the hope of awakening your own introspection, and showing what can happen when you restrain that trigger reaction to pass judgement on things you don't fully understand. Don't be so hard on yourself. Always explore possibilities to evolve into your best self, and breathe a welcome to the rest of your life.

Bibliography

Books:

Aurelius, Marcus. *Meditations*. Translated by Martin Hammond. London, UK: Penguin Classics, 2006.

Boyle, Peter, Paolo Boffetta, Albert B Lowenfels, Harry Burns, Otis Brawley, Witold Zatonski, and Jürgen Rehm, eds. *Alcohol: Science, Policy and Public Health*. Oxford: Oxford University Press, 2013.

Burroughs, William S. *Naked lunch: The Restored Text*. Edited by J. Grauerholz and B. Miles. New York, NY: Grove Press, 2001.

Geach, P Thomas. *The Virtues*. Cambridge: Cambridge University Press, 1979.

Gordon, Byron Lord George. *Don Juan*. Edited by T. G. Steffan, E. Steffan, and W. W. Pratt. London, England: Penguin Books, 1986.

Hari, Johann. *Chasing the Scream: The First and Last Days of the War on Drugs*. New York, NY: Bloomsbury Publishing, 2015.

Pray, Leslie, Ann L Yaktine, and Diana Pankevich. *Caffeine in Food and Dietary Supplements: Examining Safety: Workshop Summary*. Washington, DC: The National Academies Press, 2014.

Stanley, Debbie. *Marijuana and Your Lungs: The Incredibly Disgusting Story*. Incredibly Disgusting Drugs. New York: Rosen Pub. Group, 2000.

Stinson, Barney, and Matt Kuhn. *The Bro Code*. New York, NY: Gallery Books, 2008.

Journals:

Pizzino, Gabriele, Natasha Irrera, Mariapaola Cucinotta, Giovanni Pallio, Federica Mannino, Vincenzo Arcoraci, Francesco Squadrito, Domenica Altavilla, and Alessandra Bitto. "Oxidative Stress: Harms and Benefits for Human Health." *Oxidative medicine and cellular longevity* (2017): 1-13. https://www.ncbi.nlm.nih.gov/pmc/articles/PMC5551541/pdf/OMCL2017-8416763.pdf

Grehan, James. "Smoking and 'Early Modern' Sociability: The Great Tobacco Debate in the Ottoman Middle East (Seventeenth to Eighteenth Centuries)." *The American Historical Review* 111, no. 5 (December 2006): 1352–77. https://doi.org/10.1086/ahr.111.5.1352.

Stewart, Grace G. "A History of the Medicinal Use of Tobacco 1492–1860." *Medical History* 11, no. 3 (1967): 228–68. https://doi.org/10.1017/s0025727300012333.

Websites:

"Alcohol." World Health Organization. World Health Organization, September 21, 2008. https://www.who.int/news-room/fact-sheets/detail/alcohol.

Drugs of Abuse: A DEA Resource Guide. U.S. Department of Justice Drug Enforcement Administration, 2017. https://dev9.dea.gov/sites/default/files/drug_of_abuse.pdf.

Editors, History.com. "The Hazy History of '420'." History.com. A&E Television Networks, October 10, 2019. https://www.history.com/news/the-hazy-history-of-420.

Merrill, Sam. "George Carlin: Playboy Interview (1982)." Scraps from the loft, November 9, 2016. https://scrapsfromtheloft.com/comedy/playboy-interview-george-carlin/.

"Testimony of George Greer, M.D. in DEA Hearing on Scheduling of MDMA Under the Controlled Substances Act," April 22, 1985. https://maps.org/research-archive/dea-mdma/pdf/0065.PDF.

"Tobacco." World Health Organization, July 26, 2021. https://www.who.int/news-room/fact-sheets/detail/tobacco.

Weinreb, Michael. "The Complicated Legacy of Harry Anslinger ." Penn Stater Magazine, 2018. https://www.case.org/system/files/media/file/Penn%20Stater%20Harry%20Anslinger.pdf.

"WHO Expert Committee on Drug Dependence Critical Review: Delta-9 tetrahydrocannabinol." World Health Organization, 2018. https://cdn.who.int/media/docs/default-source/controlled-substances/thcv1.pdf?%20sfvrsn= 67f4ce3c_2&download=true

Further reading:

Feduccia, Allison A., and Michael C. Mithoefer. "MDMA-Assisted Psychotherapy for PTSD: Are Memory Reconsolidation and Fear Extinction Underlying Mechanisms?" *Progress in Neuro-Psychopharmacology and Biological Psychiatry* 84 (June 8, 2018): 221–28. https://doi.org/10.1016/j.pnpbp.2018.03.003.

Osho. *Love, Freedom, and Aloneness: The Koan of Relationships.* Edited by Sarito Carol Neiman. New York, NY: St. Martin's Griffin, 2001.

Hart, Carl L. *Drug Use for Grown-ups: Chasing Liberty in the Land of Fear.* New York, NY: Penguin Press, 2021.